IF DISNEY RAN YOUR HOSPITAL

$9\frac{1}{2}$ **Things You Would Do Differently**

BY
FRED LEE

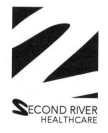

SECOND RIVER
HEALTHCARE

IF DISNEY RAN YOUR HOSPITAL
9 1/2 Things You Would Do Differently

Second River Healthcare
26 Shawnee Way, Suite C
Bozeman, MT 59715
Phone (406) 586-8775

Lee, Fred If Disney Ran Your Hospital: 9 1/2 Things You Would Do Differently
Fred Lee
p. cm.
Includes bibliographical references

ISBN-13: 978-0-9743860-0-3 (hardcover)
ISBN-13: 978-0-9743860-1-0 (softcover)
ISBN-13: 978-1-9364060-6-7 (e-Book)

1. Health services administration 2. Patient satisfaction 3. Consumer satisfaction
I. Lee, Fred   II. Title

Library of Congress control number: 2004100061

First Printing	April 2004	Seventh Printing	August 2008
Second Printing	August 2004	Eighth Printing	September 2009
Third Printing	March 2005	Ninth Printing	August 2010
Fourth Printing	August 2005	Tenth Printing	February 2012
Fifth Printing	May 2006	Eleventh Printing	October 2012
Sixth Printing	April 2007	Twelfth Printing	July 2014

Innovative Health Speakers, a speaker's bureau and division of Second River Healthcare provides a wide range of authors and nationally recognized experts for speaking events. To find out more, go to www.InnovativeHealthcareSpeakers.com or call (406) 586-8775.

Second River Healthcare books are available at special quantity discounts to use for sales promotions, employee premiums, or educational purposes. Please call for information at: 406-586-8775 or order from the websites: www.SecondRiverHealthcare.com or www.PatientLoyalty.com.

DEDICATION

To the four nurses who profoundly shaped my life through their unconditional love, and their commitment to lives of service and compassion:

To Aura, my wife, best friend, and most trusted advisor. Her encouragement keeps me motivated, and her support allows me to pursue a passion for teaching. Her talent as a caregiver, and her leadership style as a director of nurses, provides the inspiration and role model for the management principles in this book.

To Helen, my mother, who was a lifelong missionary nurse in China, setting an unwavering example of kind and selfless service.

To Margaret, the beloved mother of my daughter Stacy and son Lorin, who lost an arduous and courageous battle with encephalitis contracted when she was a school nurse in Singapore at the age of 28.

To Sylvia, my little sister, a surgical nurse, who looked up to me when I didn't deserve it and makes me feel loved and cherished as a friend and confidante.

TABLE OF CONTENTS

FOREWORD

INTRODUCTION   1

IF DISNEY RAN YOUR HOSPITAL, YOU WOULD...

CHAPTER 1	Redefine Your Competition and Focus on What Can't Be Measured	9
CHAPTER 2	Make Courtesy More Important Than Efficiency	27
CHAPTER 3	Regard Patient Satisfaction as Fool's Gold	47
CHAPTER 4	Measure to Improve, Not to Impress	67
CHAPTER 5	Decentralize the Authority to Say Yes	85
CHAPTER 6	Change the Concept of Work from Service to Theater	109
CHAPTER 7	Harness the Motivating Power of Imagination	131
CHAPTER 8	Create a Climate of Dissatisfaction	155
CHAPTER 9	Cease Using Competitive Monetary Rewards to Motivate People	173
CHAPTER 10	Close the Gap Between Knowing and Doing	193

CONCLUSION   209

FOREWORD

THREE LEVELS OF KNOWLEDGE

By Dean Hubbard
President of Northwest Missouri State University and
Former National Malcolm Baldrige Award Examiner

It gives me great pleasure to be a small part of the launching of a significant book on quality service and the culture it takes to sustain it.

Someone has said, "I am not interested in simplicity on this side of complexity. I am only interested in simplicity on the other side of complexity."

This axiom suggests that there are three stages of knowledge. The first level is simplicity born of ignorance, as when somebody says, "Oh, that's simple," but doesn't know what they are talking about. The second level is complexity born of understanding—when one realizes a subject is far more complex than it first appears on the surface. The third level is simplicity born of profound understanding. Only a few get to this lofty state. Fred Lee is among that elite group. People who know little about customer satisfaction and loyalty think it is simple. "It's just practicing the Golden Rule," they will say dismissively. Organizational leaders at this level believe they can effect change by simply elaborating on the Golden Rule with statements of mission, vision, and core values. But they quickly learn the discouraging truth that changing from a culture of "what's in it for me," to "what would be best for my customer" is impossible at that level of simplicity. When they begin to see that it is harder than it seems, some give up and make excuses for their particular organization. "We're in the inner city," they will say. Or, "Our facility needs to be modernized first." Or, "There's a labor shortage and we can't find good people anymore."

However, the best leaders redouble their efforts through exhaustive reading, learning from the great quality thinkers like Deming, Juran, and Crosby, and benchmarking other organizations. I have been on this journey at the college and university level for nearly thirty years. I know what I am talking about, and so do all the members of our leadership team. With the right thinking and relentless improvement, Northwest Missouri State University is the only educational institution to win the coveted Missouri Quality Award twice.

Sometime, stand facing the leadership shelves at Barnes and Noble and ponder this thought: Every single book in front of you, and hundreds not on display, all have something unique and important to teach about cultural transformation, human motivation, process improvement, and quality service. If one were to read them all, he or she would be overwhelmed by the complexity of creating the ideal organizational culture. What one longs for at this point is someone who can strip away the trivial and distill the essence of all this knowledge into a handful of principles born of profound understanding. That's what Fred Lee has done for hospital leadership in this immensely readable book–much of which I have found just as applicable to the university experience.

Fred Lee speaks as a keen observer of individual motivation and group participation in organizational goals. He established his career in hospital leadership and uses Disney as his benchmark because he has been inside the Disney culture as a cast member, consultant, and facilitator. What helps give his writing and speaking its most profound "simplicity on the other side of complexity" is his extensive use of personal experiences and relevant stories to demonstrate every principle he teaches. Even though he specializes in healthcare, he has been a big hit with our university staff who have been inspired by his passion and challenged by his insights. If you are still reading this foreword, I predict you have started a delightful journey through these pages.

INTRODUCTION

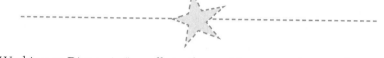

Working at Disney is "a walk in the park" compared to working in a hospital.

That's what I thought after being a Disney cast member for a short time to help develop and facilitate a program called *The Disney Approach to Quality Service for the Healthcare Industry*. Most people who have worked at Disney started there early in their lives. I had the unique privilege of being part of their organization in 1996 and 1997 after a career in hospital senior leadership and hospital service-excellence consulting and training.

Being a manager at Disney must be 10 times easier than being a clinical manager in a hospital. Frontline employees get paid about the same, but a nurse's aide has a far more difficult customer, is in an environment with far higher risks, and faces situations that cannot be standardized. At Disney, the customers start out happy and excited instead of afraid and sad. They stand in lines, but not in pain. They take a ride that is duplicated a million times, while every experience in a hospital is highly personal and unique.

The healthcare industry faces obstacles of monumental proportions. Hospitals lose money on most of their patients. Staffing shortages and under-capacity exist in virtually every community. The average American feels vulnerable to financial disaster because of inadequate or unaffordable insurance coverage. Young people are not choosing nursing as a desirable profession or hospitals as desirable places to work. Hospitals teeter on the edge of bankruptcy because of reimbursement that is constantly adjusted downward. Meanwhile the costs of drugs and technology are skyrocketing. The constant threat of malpractice suits is driving physicians out of business and creating volumes of regulations and paperwork. And this is just a partial list!

In the midst of these overwhelming problems, it is humbling to write a book on culture and leadership. It can also be demoralizing to set Disney up as an example. From where most hospital managers sit, Disney looks like a picnic compared to the fiscal, legal, and regulatory nightmare they face every day in a high-risk environment over which they have very little of the kind of control they would have at Disney.

It is my hope that the reader of this book does not think I am naive about what it is like to manage in today's hospital. The truth is, I believe it is the hardest management job in the world. I wish I could offer solutions to all the epic difficulties healthcare managers face every day, but the scope of this book is necessarily limited to those approaches that bring out the best behaviors in workers and provide the best emotional experience for patients. In this one aspect of a manager's role, made even more difficult in today's environment, I believe Disney has some insights to offer.

According to the 2002 report on *Competing for Service* from the Healthcare Advisory Board, this topic heads the list as the most requested topic for future reports. Their *1998 Report on Service Excellence* was their all-time best-seller. In the intervening years between these two reports, little if any progress has been made. In fact, national inpatient-satisfaction scores have been falling. One survey placed the IRS at number 27 and hospitals at number 28 on a list of 30 industries measured.

NOBODY HAS MOVED THE CHEESE.

Ninety percent of hospitals now have some form of patient-satisfaction survey. Most are in a regional or national database for comparative scores. What matters to patients is well known and well documented. Furthermore, these vital elements are not new and have not changed. When it comes to what the patient judges as "excellent care," it is pretty much the same today as it was 100 years ago. With all the talk about change, certain *values* and patient needs never change. When I helped develop our first patient-satisfaction survey instrument at Florida Hospital in the eighties, there was no national database, and we

were among the first to send out a survey every month to
put together a team that included Kent Seltman, our
marketing, Jo Welch, our nationally recognized patient re_
several nurses, a physician, a chaplain, and some other internal experts
to come up with the right questions to ask. The team made a list of the
things we thought mattered most to patients. Then we tried to
anticipate which half dozen or so should be weighted as being most
significant. These would become our themes for teaching patient-
focused care. Blended with a mission rooted in Christian values of
service and love, we decided on five behaviors that mattered most. If
our employees gave special attention to the following, we were sure we
would earn the loyalty of our patients.

Sense people's needs before they ask (initiative).
Help each other out (teamwork).
Acknowledge people's feelings (empathy).
Respect the dignity and privacy of everyone (courtesy).
Explain what's happening (communication).

In the passing years tens of thousands of patient-satisfaction
surveys from a score of research companies have validated these five
behaviors as having the highest correlation with overall satisfaction and
loyalty. They are values that all of us can authenticate intuitively. They
never go out of style. In 1846, Florence Nightingale wrote in her *Notes
on Nursing*, which is still assigned reading in some nursing schools,
"Apprehension, uncertainty, waiting and fear of surprise, do a patient
more harm than any exertion...Always tell a patient, and tell him
beforehand, when you are going out and when you will be back,
whether it is for a day, an hour or ten minutes."[1]

In the seventies, no less than the greatest leadership guru of all
time, Peter Drucker, produced some research that showed that the
single most important need of a patient is for "assurance." He suggested
that by focusing on the patient's need for assurance, caregivers would
be creating patient satisfaction and loyalty.

What matters most to patients is as true today as it has ever been.
To play off the title of a leading best-seller, nobody has moved the

.eese when it comes to the things that matter most to the patient.

Nobody has moved the cheese when it comes to what motivates and keeps good employees either. Much like patient satisfaction, employee satisfaction is no mystery. According to Gallup research in Buckingham and Coffman's *First, Break All the Rules*, employees leave managers, not organizations. That's nothing new. It has always been true—and true for the same reasons. Although the authors attempt to shatter some myths held by poor and average managers, the study confirms that great managers often go against many commonly held beliefs and practices to achieve high productivity and loyalty. There is nothing new, however, in *What the World's Greatest Managers Do Differently* (the book's subtitle). Great managers have always done these things, from innate and practiced talent, if not from what is commonly taught in business school.

IT'S ABOUT CULTURE, NOT SERVICE.

Someone has said, "He who knows only one culture knows none."

Constantly comparing cultures comes as naturally to me as shaking hands or bowing graciously to a guest. I am the product of two very different cultures. My American parents were both born in China of career missionaries. They lived their whole lives, except for college and retirement, in China where I was also born and raised. The infusion of Eastern and Western views on life, work, and family has been as effortless as learning to speak and think in two languages as a child.

My own career path started as a teacher, hit its stride as a senior vice president at Florida Hospital (the Disney Hospital) in Orlando, took an interesting detour through the Magic Kingdom, and has returned full circle to a life of reflection and teaching. A major influence in my thinking about patient care and how to inspire caregivers has been my wife, Aura, who was the director of nurses at Florida Hospital East Orlando for 10 years.

The experience I had as a Disney cast member was brief. Steve Heise, then manager of the Business Programs Division, heard me speak to a roomful of hospital managers on how to improve the patient experience and create an environment where caregivers love to work. At the end of the seminar, he invited me to lunch the next week and asked me to be part of a team of facilitators and program developers at Disney University. Our job was to reshape an acclaimed program *The Disney Approach to Quality Service for the Healthcare Industry*. In addition we created a new program on customer loyalty.

My academic pursuits paralleled my career path. With a master's degree in social studies I taught history and political science. While teaching, my interests and additional graduate work shifted to social psychology, which opened the door to hospital marketing and communication. As a vice president at Shawnee Mission Medical Center near Kansas City, I immersed myself in the growing trend to introduce the discipline and principles of marketing into hospital strategic planning and communication.

During one of the many seminars and courses I took in the 1980s, I wholeheartedly embraced and began to teach a concept I first heard from Terrance Rynn, a leading healthcare marketing consultant. "There is a profound difference between selling and marketing," he said. "Selling is trying to get people to want what you have. Marketing is trying to have what people want. When you have what people want, it makes selling unnecessary."

I believe a hospital's primary customer is the physician. Technically speaking, hospitals don't have patients; physicians do. Hospitals exist to take care of physicians' patients. Marketing is trying to have what physicians want. It would take an entire book to do justice to models of physician practice, partnership, and ownership, as well as their needs and wants and how to satisfy them—the subject of another book.

Employees also share many aspects with customers. Like physicians and patients, they can choose to leave and go someplace else with their skills. They can be satisfied or dissatisfied. Their loyalty is also critical in a hospital's ultimate success. Marketing is trying to have what employees want. Another entire book could be dedicated to the leadership and management skills that create a productive and positive work experience.

Terry Rynn's insight became my mantra and the driving force behind my participation in strategic planning at Florida Hospital and our efforts to market healthcare services. Whenever a department would come to me or someone in our department for "marketing ideas," they usually meant ideas for advertising and promoting what they had. I, on the other hand, wanted to understand how the service was designed and delivered, how that compared to what the competition was doing, and what the physician or patient would expect. It seemed to me that if a service was sub-par or outdated or frustrating, we should consider redesigning the service before promoting it. I believed that the worst thing you can do for a poorly delivered service is to get more physicians or patients to try it and find out how bad it is. This sometimes did not set well with department directors who viewed my marketing expertise as being limited to selling and my questions about ease of use, competitors' practices, convenience, or value-added features as needlessly intrusive.

I am still dedicated to helping hospitals *have* what people *want* instead of defending an our-way-is-the-only-way approach. I have chosen to write largely about patient needs, wants, and expectations. When patients are pleased with their hospitalization, so are their physicians, and to a great extent, so are caregivers. And in my experience, nobody designs and trains around individual customer needs and wants better than the Disney organization. This book represents my reflections on and comparisons with these two cultures.

THIS IS A DIFFERENT BOOK ABOUT DISNEY.

Although I was intimately involved in the content of *The Disney Approach to Quality Service* and was a facilitator for the program, this book is not a rehash of that material. Readers who have attended the seminar at Disney University will find the themes of this book significantly different and, I hope, much more thought-provoking and powerful.

I am also not interested in repeating what many of the books and articles on the "Disney Way" have already written about to the point of cliché, such as Disney's attention to detail, hiring right, on-stage/off-stage behaviors, walking the talk, making everything fit a theme, calling customers "guests" and employees "cast members," etc. Most of these things have little, if anything, to do with deep change. They are fairly superficial and easily implemented. I have found from extensive experience, however, that such things have done little to improve the perceptions of hospital patients.

I have written ten chapters on things Disney does differently, but the first chapter is more fundamental and less innovative to most readers than the rest, so I have decided to subtitle this book, *9 1/2 Things You Would Do Differently*. Also, the number 10 has a ring of finality or completeness to it that I do not intend to imply. Obviously Disney does many more things, even significant things, differently from hospitals. These are simply the ones that most influenced my thinking because they are more about culture than about strategy or implementation. I believe that any healthcare team can find its own way to greatness if it has the passion and competence to do so. In addition it helps to have clarity about what's important, which approaches work, and which approaches do not work in building a committed culture. My role is to help hospital managers initiate the right conversations about the right things with the right people by using themes I found particularly insightful at Disney back in 1996.

Although this book was written with hospital managers in mind it should also be appealing to staff at all levels. It is filled with personal examples and stories that I hope will stimulate conversations on creating the ideal patient experience. It is fairly comprehensive and includes what I believe are the principles most likely to improve patient perceptions. It reflects what I hope is a deeper approach to clinical practices by focusing on ways of thinking rather than prescribing actions to implement. Action follows thought, and if our thinking is changed we will find the ways to create a culture that inspires caregivers and reshapes the patient's experience toward a more trusting and compassionate environment for healing to take place.

Finally, I write about Disney because that is the culture that piqued my curiosity, where I had first-hand experience. Had I worked at Marriott or Southwest Airlines, or any number of other world-class organizations, I might have chosen one of them as my model. Using Disney does not mean I think Disney is unsurpassed in cultural excellence.

---

1. Florence Nightingale, *Notes on Nursing: What It Is and What It Is Not* (New York: D. Appleton-Century Company, 1946) p. 38.

Chapter 1 Redefine your Competition and Focus on What Can't Be Measured

Let's start with the most self-evident theme in this book. This chapter is the "1/2 thing" alluded to in the title of the book because it has more to do with what we already know than with new concepts. It reminds us of a fundamental frame of reference rather than actual changes that must be made. In the subsequent chapters of this book, the principles require important shifts in thinking as well as sustained, committed effort. This does not minimize the content of this chapter. Indeed these basic principles underlie the entire book, and clarity on them, which is often lacking in the hospitals I have visited, is imperative for a manager to lead effectively.

At Florida Hospital, where I was vice president for strategic planning and marketing, employees have taken great pride through the years in the belief that they worked for the "best" hospital in central Florida. We knew people could choose one of our competitor hospitals. When Disney chose Florida Hospital to be their healthcare provider, it seemed to confirm our view that we were winning against our competition. The pride generated by this belief was palpable throughout the organization. It didn't matter if we had scientific proof or not. We were the best because we believed the community thought so, and so did Disney.

Later, when I worked at the Disney Institute, I learned to think differently about our competition. I was sitting in Disney Traditions, the three-day orientation program for all new employees. Our teacher was a young man whose regular job was working at the Jungle Cruise attraction. He looked at the roomful of expectant, eager faces and asked the question, "Who is Disney's competition?" Since good responses got a little toy character tossed to one of us, we were quick to name some of central Florida's major attractions: Universal Studios, Cypress Gardens, Church Street Station, Cape Canaveral, the beaches, even Busch Gardens in Tampa. Our instructor wrote each of these on a flip chart. When we could no longer think of any more, he looked all around the room, then at his flip chart, and dramatically crossed out all our responses. "At Disney we take a much larger view of competition. The truth is that our competition is anyone our customers compare us to."

The same thing is true for a hospital. Clinical outcomes can be measured, and these numbers can be compared to measures of clinical quality at other hospitals. Hospitals make these comparisons all the time to determine best clinical practices. But most patients do not. They hold in their minds a mental picture of how a person should be treated, and that picture becomes the standard by which their experience is judged.

KNOW THE FIELD OF BATTLE FOR THE CUSTOMER'S MIND.

It is only natural that to a physician, administrator, or clinician, quality is primarily judged by clinical outcomes. And rightly so. What isn't so obvious is that the satisfaction and loyalty of their customers are not primarily won on the field of who has the best clinical quality, any more than airlines win the loyalty of their customers on the field of who has the best safety record. Most airlines have about the same safety records. And most clinical outcomes are viewed by patients as the purview of their physician who would not put them in the hands of incompetent people or an unsafe environment. When there is a plane crash, an airline will suffer a major setback in public opinion, just as a hospital suffers when a preventable tragedy occurs in its operating

room. But precluding such a catastrophe, patients j   ‍o
experience by the way they are treated as a person, not by t
are treated for their disease. Figure 1.1 includes a list of th
from inpatient-satisfaction surveys that have the highest correlation
between likelihood to recommend and overall satisfaction with their
hospital. Notice how the questions with the highest correlation are
mostly from perceptions about how one is treated as a person, not
clinical competencies.

Figure 1.1: Top Drivers of Patient Satisfaction

Press Ganey Associates: Top 10 Drivers of Patient Satisfaction
Mail-in survey questions (out of 48) that correlate most highly
with "likely to recommend"

1. How well staff worked together to care for you	.79
2. Overall cheerfulness of the hospital	.74
3. Response to concerns/complaints made during your stay	.68
4. Amount of attention paid to your personal and special needs	.65
5. Staff sensitivity to the inconvenience of hospitalization	.65
6. How well nurses kept you informed	.64
7. Staff's effort to include you in decisions about your treatment	.64
8. Nurses attitude toward your requests	.64
9. Skill of the nurses	.63
10. Friendliness of the nurses	.62

Press, Ganey *Satisfaction Report*, August, 2003

Gallup: Top Seven Drivers of Patient Satisfaction
Telephone survey questions (out of 27) that correlate most highly
with "overall satisfaction"

1. Nurses anticipated your needs.	.64
2. Staff and departments worked together as a team.	.64
3. Staff responded with care and compassion.	.62
4. Staff advised you if there were going to be delays.	.61
5. Nurses explained about medications, procedures, and routines.	.60
6. Nurses responded promptly to pain management.	.60
7. Nurses responded in a reasonable amount of time.	.60

The Gallup Organization, 1999

In the battle for the supremacy of perceptions in the patient's mind, our
competition is anyone the patient compares us to. Unfortunately they
do not usually compare us to other hospitals. People don't make an
exception by saying, "Compared to other nurses she's okay but she
couldn't cut it as a waitress or any other service provider." Nine out

ten of the top drivers of satisfaction could apply to how a person is treated anywhere. Only one in ten is hospital specific. After many years of collecting data on patient satisfaction and loyalty, we now know quantitatively what we have always known intuitively—patients reserve their good word of mouth and loyalty for hospitals where they feel their needs were anticipated and met by a courteous, caring staff. When one reads through this list of top drivers of patient satisfaction and loyalty from two of the largest organizations that do hospital surveys, it is clear that often what hospital managers focus on, namely clinical and process outcomes, is not where the battle for the consumer's mind is being waged.

When hospitals spend most of their efforts in clinical results and process improvement, their data are defined by *outcomes* and therefore can be measured objectively. The *patient*, however, judges quality by his or her *perceptions*, something that is subjective and cannot be verified in the same way as outcomes. The patient is judging the overall *experience* of being in a hospital. It frequently comes as a surprise to hospital personnel when the clinical outcomes are excellent but the patient is displeased or angry. Both of these concepts—perceptions and outcomes—are vital, but each has a vastly different impact on hospital viability and success, as shown in Figure 1.2.

Figure 1.2: The Economic Impact of Performance Improvement

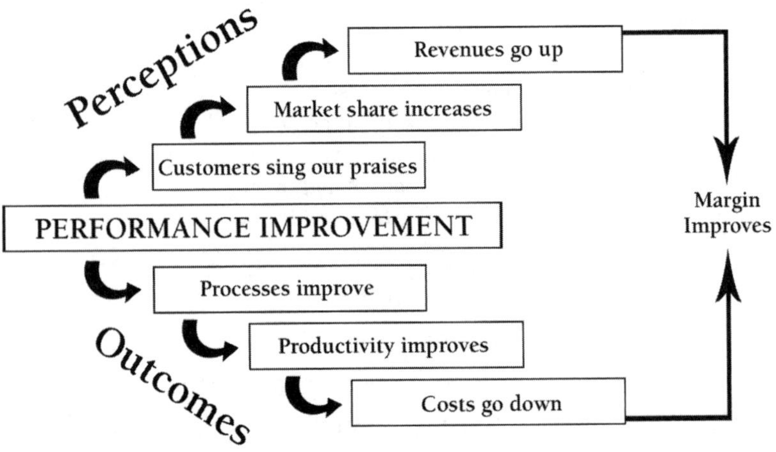

IT TAKES A DIFFERENT SKILL SET TO MANAGE PERCEPTIONS.

The engine for growth is patient perceptions. The engine for efficiency is process improvement. If we are going to create a culture where employees take an active part in helping sustain the company, this should be common knowledge throughout the organization. Off the top of their heads, every caregiver ought to be able to list the top three or four drivers of patient perceptions that produce loyalty. Every manager of a unit that has patient contact should be focusing regularly on these top drivers and requiring staff to be proficient in ways that create the key impressions that matter most to patients. How to shape these perceptions and manage them effectively is vastly different from approaches and techniques for improving outcomes (see Figure 1.3).

Figure 1.3: Improving Outcomes and Perceptions

To Improve...

Outcomes	Perceptions
Focus on team responsibility	Focus on personal responsibility
Map and study processes	Take action on information—just do it
Understand process variation	Understand patient perceptions
Improve staff competence & skills	Improve staff behaviors & attitudes
Stress what people should be doing	Stress what people should be saying
Seek measurable results	Seek to impact impressions
"Zero defects" thinking	"Best possible" thinking
Eliminate carelessness	Eliminate avoidance

The first thing to have clear is that outcomes are delivered by teams, whereas impressions are delivered by individuals. Managing each of these realities takes a different skill set. Most clinical managers are not equally gifted at doing both. But with more understanding of their essential differences and subsequent different approaches, any determined manager can become proficient at both. For process improvement, it takes many people in many roles to create an efficient team. Changing one part of a process can dramatically change another part of the process in unintended ways. To make sure we see the entire process, cross-functional teams often start by mapping and studying the steps in a process by which work gets completed. Then with the help of statistical graphs and numerical data, bottlenecks and redundancy can be spotted and fixed. An entire course of training in facilitating process improvement is standard in most large hospitals. These principles and techniques are particularly exciting to the analytical mind.

However, impressions are created by individuals in one-on-one interactions. Managers who like to deal with everything in a team setting while taking an analytical approach to problem solving, will often fail in this arena. Their natural inclination will be to admonish an entire staff in a staff meeting for inappropriate behavior by one member of the group. They think they are serving the needs of the group by sharing something everyone needs to understand, but the person who created the problem is not likely to recognize himself or herself in the admonition. There is no substitute for dealing with the offender directly, whether it's about poor attitude, inappropriate dress, language, or demeanor. Not to do so is seen as a sign of weakness on the part of the manager and causes resentment by the rest of the team. In fact "wimpy managers" is often cited by subordinates as their biggest grievance with a manager they do not respect. It takes much more courage to rebuke a staff member in private than to lecture an entire group about what everybody should be doing and hoping the offender gets the message.

For improving outcomes, the focus is on what people *do*. Are they doing it right? Are they following sterile technique? Are they knocking before entering a room? Are they answering the call lights in the amount of time that has been set as a standard? Are they getting important information on the charts in the right place? Are they checking wristbands?

However, when it comes to perceptions, it's what a person *says* or *doesn't say* that creates the impression. For instance, let's take an item that was number one on the Press Ganey survey for nearly a decade (now number 12): "Staff's concern for your privacy." Hospitals found that they could not seem to improve this perception no matter how hard they tried to protect the patient's privacy. They taught staff to do things like knocking before entering, drawing the curtain,

protecting patient confidentiality, closing the patient's doo
noisy, and covering exposed parts of the body. But it was w.
started to focus on the key word in the question
"concern"–that they made progress. They began to ask th   ....on,
"How do we give the *impression* that we are genuinely *concerned* for their
privacy?" People do not notice concern unless we say something. A
nurse may close the door and draw the curtain and begin a procedure,
thinking everything has been done to protect the patient's privacy. But
it is only when the nurse says something like "I'm here to give you a
bath, and just to make sure nobody barges in on us I have closed the
door and I am going to pull your curtain too," that she creates the
impression that she is concerned about the patient.

Or let's say that there is a lot of commotion at the nurses' station
late at night giving report to the next shift. A nurse quickly closes the
patient's door out of concern for the patient's privacy. Yet the patient
probably thinks, *Why are they closing my door? I'll bet they're talking about
me.* The way to create the impression of concern is to say something to
the patient like "Mr. Lee, would you like your door closed? We get
pretty noisy out here while we're giving report. It shouldn't last much
longer." Only by concentrating on what is *said* while doing something
did hospitals begin to see significant improvement in patient
perceptions that staff showed concern for patient privacy.

Six Sigma, the process improvement certification program so
popular in manufacturing, has also made it into hospitals as the latest
iteration of the quality movement. Essentially it seeks a "zero defect"
environment and refines outcome measurements. This can
significantly reduce mistakes like medication errors, but as a roadmap
for patient satisfaction and loyalty a "zero defect" approach is useless.
How do you determine a "defect" in human communication with all the
subtleties of body language, facial expression and tone of voice? We
might be able to say we have "no tolerance" for rudeness, but rudeness
is rarely the reason someone misses an opportunity for courtesy or
compassion. Anyway, zero tolerance for rudeness is not a standard for
behavior that wins friends and supporters. How do you score missed
opportunities? How do you count the ways in which acceptable
communication could have been better? How do you measure thi

warmth, cheerfulness (number 2 on the Press Ganey list), and friendliness? They have a huge impact on perceptions, but can you standardize them in such a way as to be able to spot the "defect?" Of course not. Here our thinking needs to be "best possible."

Clinical competencies are tested all the time in hospitals to make sure that anyone assigned to a piece of equipment or procedure knows how to do it exactly as prescribed. But the enemy of competence is not incompetence; it's carelessness. We make sure safety inspections are built in to our systems as back up checks in case someone is careless. When a serious clinical mistake is made resulting in a malpractice lawsuit, it is not usually because someone was incompetent. It is far more likely to be a case where a perfectly competent person was careless and our system of checks failed to catch it.

In the same way, we can say that rudeness is not the enemy of courtesy. A perceived lack of cheerfulness, friendliness, or caring (the high-impact words found in our surveys) is not generally the result of rudeness or even indifference on the part of uncaring, unhappy people. It is usually because a cheerful, caring person did not look up, missed the opportunity to connect, make eye contact, or become aware of the patient's feelings. I would call this avoidance, not rudeness or indifference. If you are the manager of a department where customer perceptions are important, stop concentrating on "mistakes" like rudeness, and set a standard related to avoidance. If I ran a hospital, I would have the same standard that Disney has. You never pass another individual in the hallways without greeting that person with a smile. I would expect every manager to role model that behavior and require it of everyone in the department. Avoidance must be considered a violation of the organization's culture, because with each avoidance we have a missed opportunity for the little courtesies that add up to an overall perception of a cheerful, friendly place.

CULTURE TRUMPS STRATEGY.

The first thing I learned at Disney, along with everyone else who
h you must do even if you have been offered a position),
s joining a culture, not getting a job. This was impressed
e I turned in my application. All of us applicants were

required to view a video before handing in the forms we had filled out. The film started out with Disney terminology, like employees are called "cast members" and customers are called "guests." Enthusiastic cast members spoke excitedly of how much fun it was to work at Disney. But before the film had ended they described what would be expected of you if you chose to work there. They told us that we would be expected to be "aggressively friendly" and greet all cast members by name. This was not difficult because every cast member's badge had his or her first name in large print, which could be read from at least twenty feet. Then there was a section on "appearance guidelines" which spelled out the way we were expected to dress. No facial hair for men; no frosted hair or conspicuous makeup for women—things like that. Later I learned that about 15% of applicants throw their applications away after viewing the film. Obviously not everybody wants to be part of a culture where such behaviors are cultural expectations.

Someone once observed that, "Culture eats strategy for lunch every day of the week." I know exactly what that means, especially after a stint at Disney. Since I have been making the point in this chapter that what we say makes a bigger impression than what we do, we might say that our *strategy* is to teach people what to say to make the best possible impression. We might even follow up our strategy by putting a committee together to write scripts that tell people what to say in certain repetitive situations. Then we might go so far as to teach our scripts to everybody and insist that they use them. Using this line of thought, let me show you how culture sinks strategy.

Let's take the example of the top driver on the Press Ganey survey of patient perceptions, which is also at the top of the Gallup survey. They are perceptions about teamwork. We start with our question: "What can we say that gives the impression that we work together as a team?" Remember that when it comes to perceptions we are not dealing with reality, only impressions. So we come up with a script that requires every person to say, "Is there anything else you need?" before leaving a patient anytime anywhere. If the patient needs something that you cannot provide you will say, "I will tell your nurse." That's our strategy. Everybody learns it. Everybody does it. And it's guaranteed to give the impression that we "anticipate your needs" and "work together as a team."

However, there's a good chance the culture will sink this strategy in all but the most focused of patient care environments. How? Well, let's say Susan is a new housekeeper. She has been taught our script. During her first day on the job she says, "Mr. Lee, is there anything I have missed?" (A good script for housekeepers, by the way.) And then she adds, "Is there anything you need before I leave?" Mr. Lee says he needs his urinal emptied. She responds with the script, "Let me get your nurse." Then Susan walks out into the nursing culture and presents Mr. Lee's problem to a nurse. But the nurse appears irritated (one of those agency nurses, no doubt, who missed our training) and snaps, "I'm too busy right now. Mr. Lee has a call button you know." Do you believe Susan will continue to practice her script if the nursing culture does not seem to appreciate her interruptions? Not likely.

The real question is: Will our culture support our strategies? Once we get this in mind, we realize that whatever scripts we teach people to say to patients need to be followed up by cultural expectations that are equally rehearsed. That's how a good hospital can become a great hospital in patient perceptions.

What would be the result in this example if the culture is one where all nurses treat housekeepers, and everyone else from other departments, as valued members of the health care team? What could we teach them that would inspire that? Well, let's back up to the point where Susan speaks to the nurse, and develop this sample script further and see what it can do for the culture.

Susan: I was just in Mr. Lee's room and he needs his urinal emptied.
Nurse: Hi. I'm Janet. I don't think I have seen you before."
Susan: Hi. I'm Susan from housekeeping. This is my first day.
Nurse: (smiling) Well, welcome to our unit, Susan. This is a great unit. I hope we make you feel welcome working here. Now what was it Mr. Lee needed?
Susan: His urinal emptied.
Nurse: Thank you for telling me. We need all the eyes and ears we can get around here. It was nice meeting you, Susan.

Obviously I do not mean that these exact words be use only that the sentiment of appreciation for the h departments gets communicated any time someone sh need. If it does, do you think Susan will continue to take paue.. concerns to the nurses? Of course she will, because the culture supports her when she does.

But we can still improve this scene in an important way by going a bit deeper. Remember the purpose is to create the perception that we "work together as a team." Why not instruct the nurse to say something like this when she enters Mr. Lee's room:

Nurse: Susan told me you needed your urinal emptied.
Mr. Lee: Susan?
Nurse: Yes, the housekeeper who was just here. She told me.
Mr. Lee: Oh, yes.
Nurse: (while taking the urinal) Did you know today was Susan's first day? Seems like a nice person, don't you think?

When Press Ganey sends a questionnaire or Gallup calls Mr. Lee and asks, "How well did the staff work together to care for you?" what impression will Mr. Lee remember? He will probably remember how a housekeeper took his needs to the nurse, who obviously must like housekeepers because she knew her name and spoke nicely about her. What that nurse said to the housekeeper and Mr. Lee turns out to have the biggest impact on his perceptions, not the simple question, "Is there anything else you need, I have the time."

Sidebar: I threw the last phrase in because it is common to teach it in hospitals in order to create the impression that nurses are not too busy to care for patients. However, anything that is a little out of the ordinary begins to lose spontaneity and not sound normal. It will never sound contrived or forced to say some phrases over and over, like "good morning," "thank you" and "you're welcome." But a phrase like, "I have the time," said by every single person begins to sound overly rehearsed and insincere. I think it should only be said when it fits a certain situation like when a nurse drops into the patient's room unexpectedly and says, "You haven't called me in a while. Do you need anything? I have the time right now."

We could easily take every item on a survey and drill down from ور scripts into the culture and do exactly as I have done with this one item. It would be well worth the time to have the conversations that lead us to scrutinize our cultures, and hone our appreciation skills, especially if we are passionate about creating positive patient perceptions.

FOCUSING ON COMPLAINTS
WILL MISS WHAT MATTERS MOST.

Many managers assume that if they don't get many complaints they are doing fine–and that if they focus on complaints, they will be dealing with the issues that matter most to patients. This comes from the process mind-set, where a process is working well if there are no complaints. But for perceptions, focusing on complaints does little, if anything, to improve overall patient loyalty. Let's return to the top drivers of patient satisfaction and loyalty in the Press Ganey survey (Figure 1.1). A question that is conspicuous by its absence in these top 10 factors is anything about food. This is especially interesting because in most hospitals more complaints are received about the food than any other item. But the striking fact is that the quality of the food has the lowest correlation coefficient of the 48 questions in the survey except for temperature of the room.

Focusing on what gets the most complaints is not focusing on what is most important in creating the impressions by which patients judge their care. It is conceivable that a hospital, by hiring a prominent chef, could get terrific scores for food quality and see no rise in their overall satisfaction scores. Conversely, a hospital might get abysmal scores on the food and maintain high levels of patient loyalty. Why is this? There are several reasons:

1. People complain about things that can be verified objectively. But as we have seen, what can be measured objectively does not correlate as highly with overall satisfaction as the kinds of things that are purely subjective.

2. People do not complain about people's attitudes, the leading correlation with overall satisfaction. Only if someone is outright rude, might hospitals hear about it–even when the patient is asked.

3. People complain within the scope of what is conventionally expected. They do not mention what behavior would win their loyalty because it would be behavior that is beyond what they could reasonably expect.

4. Only four out of 100 dissatisfied customers will complain, according to research conducted by the Technical Assistance Research Program.

5. Getting a person to complain about something like a nurse's attitude is almost impossible while they are in the hospital because nobody wants to get into a "he-said, she-said" showdown with a clinical worker, especially when they could retaliate by ignoring the patient.

6. Most customers do not believe complaining will do any good. Since they can punish your organization invisibly by negative word of mouth, they won't stick their necks out to let you know their true feelings.

To raise patient satisfaction scores, to get patient loyalty, a hospital's best strategy is to focus on the things that most correlate with overall satisfaction, even if they get no complaints in those categories. This means getting extra good at hiring cheerful, empathetic people where they must interact with patients. It means teaching caregivers to actively solicit the needs of patients. It means teaching nurses to say something that shows they are concerned about a patient's privacy when preparing for an immodest procedure. It means stressing the importance to all personnel of constantly briefing the patient on the status of his or her condition, delays, tests, treatments, and what medications are for. It means making sure everyone knows how to defuse the anger and regain the goodwill of an irate patient or family member. It means taking an active interest in the whole family and helping them feel they are part of the healing team. It means valuing the gift of empathy, instead of considering professional distance our standard for bedside caring. It means teaching the importance of all these things that patients do *not* complain about, but that dramatically affect their emotional state and consequently their feelings of loyalty.

DISNEY IS YOUR COMPETITOR.

Now let's go back to the title of this chapter about redefining the competition. As long as we define our competition only in terms of our product, namely superior clinical outcomes, we will see our competition as other hospitals that are doing no better or worse than we are. That thinking breeds a false sense of security since, as we have seen, patients judge us along very different quality dimensions than we judge ourselves.

If Disney ran your hospital, you would define your competition for customer loyalty as *anyone the customer compares you to*. And for every patient or family that has been to Disney, Disney has slipped into their minds and become your competition. How many of your patients work at service organizations where they have been highly trained in service excellence? How do you stack up in the minds of those people? It may seem unfair, but the reality is that what matters most to a patient in the hospital is the same thing that matters most to a family at Disney. If you lived in Orlando, you would feel it.

Not long ago I received a letter from the chief of police in Altamonte Springs, a suburb of Orlando where I live. I had recently been issued a traffic citation for speeding, and I was sure this was a letter informing me that I could not sign up for a third time to take the remedial driving class in order to get points taken off my record. I opened the letter and this is what it said:

> Dear Mr. Lee:
>
> On September 7, you had contact with our police officer(s) in reference to a traffic violation.
>
> Our agency is concerned with its image with the public. We are seeking your assistance.
>
> Enclosed you will find a request for information. It would be appreciated if you would answer the questions and return it. The postage has been paid.
>
> With your help, we will be better able to assess our personnel and how they function.
>
> Sincerely,
> William A. Liquori
> Chief of Police

The form attached to the letter had the badge number of a police officer at the top and these questions. After each question were several lines where the respondent could write comments and further space on the back of the form for lengthy explanations:

1. Was the officer professional? Yes __ No __
2. Were you treated with respect? Yes __ No __
3. Were you treated fairly? Yes __ No __
4. Do you feel the situation was handled properly? Yes __ No __
5. Understanding that this may have been a difficult situation, were you generally satisfied with the Altamonte Springs Police Department? Yes __ No

Only in Orlando, I thought as I read this letter and feedback form. *Look how Disney has raised the bar in service and courtesy for everybody in Orlando. Even the police can't escape the influence of Disney!*

Nearly everyone who lives in central Florida has been to Disney. They have experienced quality service and know what it feels like. It is not surprising that to compete in service in Orlando, you had better be as good as Disney. What is surprising is that the police–who are a monopoly and work for the state, not a private enterprise–act as if they are competing in the service sector. This takes an administrator who recognizes that their reputation is in the hands of the community and that the community judges a police officer's behavior every bit as critically as they do a ticket taker who works at Disney. If you ask a group of police officers, as I once did, who their customer is, most of them would probably say, "Society is our customer, not the guy who is breaking the law. We are here to protect society from dangerous drivers. Lawbreakers are not customers. When we give someone a ticket, we are not performing a service for that person."

This reminds me a bit of the early days of guest relations in hospitals. I often heard variations on the theme that "we have patients, not customers, and this is not Disney."

A police officer could say, "There's nothing nice about giving a ticket to someone. I have to care about society. I can't be concerned about how the violator feels." But in Altamonte Springs there is a chief of police who believes the customer is any member of the community whose word of mouth can influence how the police are perceived. As a member of society, the violator of a traffic ordinance is still a person whose opinion about the police matters. He deserves courtesy and respect every bit as much as he would deserve it as a customer of a restaurant or hotel. Police who take this view are practicing the understanding that their reputation is based on the adage in this chapter—*anyone the customer compares them to.*

ONE MORE TIME—
IT'S ABOUT IMPRESSIONS, NOT REALITY.

Notice that whether we work together as a team or not is an impression we create in the patient's mind. It is possible we are working great as a team but leave the impression that we are not. Or we could have terrible teamwork in reality yet leave the impression that we work as a team. The two are not synonymous. The police chief who had me evaluate his officer was focused on the *impression* his officers were making on the community, not on service excellence per se.

Once I was working with a group of transporters in a hospital. One of the young men confided to me, "I never have a problem with angry patients that have been waiting a long time for a transporter. You know what I do?" he said. "I always start to run with my empty wheelchair just before I turn the corner that takes me into the lobby. It gives the impression that I am hurrying as fast as I can go. When people think I am doing my best to get there, they are much nicer."

When Jan Carlzon, president of Scandinavian Airlines, made the spectacular turnaround in his industry that became a model in so many management books at the start of the customer revolution, he coined the phrase "moments of truth." He defined these moments as any interaction that creates a negative or positive impression in the mind of a customer about your organization. He was, in effect, defining the competition as anyone your customer compares you to in any given interaction with a member of your staff.

If Disney ran your hospital, your nurses would begin to believe that they are judged not so much against the standard of other nurses in similar settings, but against the standards set by the nicest people giving services anywhere. And the same would be true of your housekeepers, telephone operators, managers, and physicians.

Chapter 2

Make Courtesy More Important Than Efficiency

In a busy hospital, where employees are stretched to the limit and then some, there is often a natural resistance, even outright opposition to a "service message" from top management. "This isn't Disney, and we aren't actors," they'll say. "Give us more staff and maybe we'll be able to give better service."

During my two days in Disney Traditions, our instructor asked the question, "What is the primary focus of every cast member at Disney?"

We quickly answered with variations on the concepts of courtesy and customer service. But we were wrong. "The primary focus of every cast member is safety," said our instructor. "Every one of you must be constantly aware of guest safety. If you see a child climbing over a fence, you drop everything else you are doing and stop that potentially hazardous activity. If somebody falls down or faints, rush to their aid. Nothing at Disney is more important than safety."

The instructor went on to explain that even though safety is our number one concern, the guest will not give us credit for that. At the end of the day, he told us, nobody is going to look back on their Disney experience and say, "Wow! What a safe place that was!" A safe experience is something nobody notices. Only when things do not seem safe do customers notice. So if we all do our job, the thing we are focused on is the thing that will not earn us any credit from our guests.

"There are four areas of constant quality focus at Disney," he continued, "and each of these has an order of priority. When you are faced with two conflicting demands, understanding these priorities will help you know exactly which concern takes precedence."

He then put up a poster with these four priorities in this order:

1. SAFETY
2. COURTESY
3. SHOW
4. EFFICIENCY

Safety and courtesy and efficiency are clear enough. Show, at Disney, relates to everything that makes a sensory impression. It means how well an area "shows" to the guest. For front line cast members, it refers especially to their personal appearance and how neat and clean every area of the park looks (shows).

What first struck me when I saw this list, was that their highest priority was the same as ours. In fact the criteria for admission to and discharge from a hospital is mostly about safety. If patients cannot be safe in any other setting, we admit them. When they can be safe somewhere else, we discharge them, either to a less intensive rehabilitation unit, or home. So when nurses and clinicians think we have a different primary focus from Disney's, it really isn't true.

However, that's where the similarity ends. It is putting courtesy second only to safety that is not as common in most hospitals. At most hospitals, it is not clear what comes next. Everything is given equal lip service, but nothing is given priority over the other. This leaves room for a lot of confusion and a great deal of variation in courtesy.

DISNEY USES AN ELEGANT LADDER INSTEAD OF PILLARS.

It is popular in hospitals to speak of their "pillars"–the four or five (I have seen as many as nine) areas of strategic focus. Pillars provide a useful model for making assignments on a strategic plan at the top of the organization. You can put each of your pillars in the hands of a person or committee to develop the goals, objectives and activities that will be necessary to carry out the plan. But as a behavioral model for organizational culture, or employee performance, pillars are not as clear as Disney's ladder of priorities. When an employee is faced with a cultural dilemma like, "should I do this or should I do that right now," it is almost always a dilemma because the employee is faced with two or more competing values—equally held by the organization. If he does the one thing, he could be in trouble for not doing the other, no matter which he chooses.

The value of Disney's ladder of priorities was immediately clear to me as I sat in Disney Traditions. What was not so clear to me then, but has since become quite profound with time, is the elegance of the particular rungs chosen for Disney's ladder.

According to the scientific method, for a theory or model to be considered "elegant" it must have clarity, simplicity, and completeness. Disney's ladder of priorities has all three. First, each of the concepts is discrete and clear. The words chosen are unambiguous and there is no fuzzy overlap in meaning between them. Secondly, the prioritizing eliminates confusion about expectations when equally good alternatives confront the chooser. Thirdly, it is complete, because it defies the observer to find any conflict of interest that is not settled by the words and priorities chosen on the ladder. Let's contrast what I am trying to say with one of the more popular pillar models in the hospital lexicon:

SERVICE PEOPLE QUALITY FINANCIAL GROWTH

To a front line employee what is the difference between service and people, or service and quality, for that matter? Does there not seem to also be some fuzzy overlap at first glance between financial and growth? Where is anything about safety? What about processes, the engine for efficiency? Where is teamwork, a vital part of process improvement and quality? If they are all a part of quality, then too much appears to be captured under quality, and probably too little under growth.

How does a front line caregiver distinguish clearly between these values by the words we have chosen? They may be useful, as I said, to delegate authority from the top for planning purposes, or even balanced scorecards, but putting these words up in front of workers tells them very little about our expectations from them. I have seen trainers try to present these pillars to front line staff, carefully explaining what is meant by each one. But I have also noticed that the people in the room are quite simply bored, because they have no idea how to apply these high-level abstractions to their daily activities and real-life choices. If everything we advocate has equal weight, how useful is listing them, or how sure are we that our list is complete?

By contrast, every eye is intent and every mind engaged when cast members are presented with the Disney ladder of priorities. They are discrete behavioral guidelines captured in one word, not a mixture of concrete and abstract ideas. Nothing tells you how to succeed at Disney as clearly as this model does. For any cast member who is looking to measure up to the expectations in a new culture, here is the key. Since we all make dozens of choices every day, every single person is eager for clarity on priorities in making those choices. By adding some vivid illustrations, Disney is able to make it clear that there is a logic to the ladder.

While we may share Disney's highest priority–safety–how do you think most hospital employees would choose to act when there is conflict between courtesy and efficiency? I would say they get the clear message by practice, whether it is the written message or not. Efficiency trumps courtesy most of the time. So, if we have made a case for the fact that our patients judge their stay by courtesy, and employees are managed according to efficiency, is there any wonder why we are making so little progress in the drive for patient satisfaction and loyalty? If courtesy is not more important than something else, it is not more important than anything. And if it is not more important than anything else by practice, why are we hammering them to be more courteous and service-minded? That puts employees in conflict everyday with what they see from leadership, and the way they are managed and held accountable by their supervisors. Such double-bind messages are destructive of the work spirit to say nothing of the shared culture.

If Disney ran your hospital, you would make courtesy more important than efficiency. By making courtesy more important than

efficiency, you would be putting corporate values in line with ∖
patients have indicated as the key drivers of their satisfaction anᴄ
loyalty. It's doubtful that higher levels of customer satisfaction and
loyalty can be achieved in any hospital that does not change its
priorities by making courtesy more important than efficiency. And this
includes the satisfaction of internal customers as well.

When I present this concept to health care audiences, I often see
what I would call guarded assent. It is as if they have been persuaded,
but have no idea how it would change anything they are currently
doing. It is one thing to buy into this principle, it's quite another thing
to know what to do with it in day-to-day operations. Because of this, I
have found it necessary to provide a number of illustrations to prime
our mental pump, so that change can flow from the well of our deepest
commitments and the soul of our passions, instead of dribbling out in
little spurts here and there, desperately trying to balance competing
values.

I GET A PERSONAL LESSON
IN COURTESY AND EFFICIENCY.

My first wake-up call in customer service occurred in the late seventies,
when I became vice president for marketing and development at
Shawnee Mission Medical Center near Kansas City, Missouri. My boss,
Tom Flynn, thought I should take a time-management course offered in
a fine hotel in downtown Kansas City. I went and dutifully took notes,
writing down every piece of information on managing my time. The
speaker made a special point that our secretary should screen all our
calls. This would allow us to decide if we wanted to take the call or not,
and, if so, we could prepare for the subject at hand and maybe pull out
a file to be ready with our notes. If not, we could signal the secretary to
indicate we were unavailable and would call them back later.

I returned to the office invigorated. I cleared all the clutter off my
desk. I made a resolution to handle each piece of paper only once. I
began my master to-do list. I told my secretary how to screen my calls
by asking for the caller's name and whether I knew what the call was
"in reference to."

after that we asked Ray Guthrie, the president of Overland nk, to be chairman of the hospital's foundation board. ed, we were elated to have such a powerful community us raise funds to relocate and expand our infant development center.

I will never forget the first time I placed a call to Mr. Guthrie to go over the agenda for our next foundation board meeting. I dialed the bank's main number and said, "Ray Guthrie, please," to the operator. I was expecting to get Mr. Guthrie's secretary, of course, so was surprised when he picked up the phone himself. A bit flustered, I blurted out, "Ray, this is Fred Lee from Shawnee Mission Medical Center. I was expecting to get your secretary."

"She's here," he answered. "Do you want to speak to her?"

Later on I asked Mr. Guthrie if he always took his own calls directly from the operator, or was that a fluke when I called. "Oh, no," he said. "If my door is open, my secretary lets me take all my own calls."

"But I was just in a time-management course for executives that taught us to have our secretaries screen all our calls. It's supposed to be more efficient if you do that," I said.

"Whose time is more important, yours or the caller's," he asked rhetorically.

I thought about what would happen if Ray Guthrie tried to get me on the phone by asking the operator for Fred Lee. "Is that a patient?" she would probably ask, since I was quite new to the organization. After being told that I was a vice president, she would have put him through to the executive offices, and the receptionist would have probably said, "No, Mr. Lee's office is not here. He is in the marketing and development office. Let me see if I can transfer you. By the way, if you get cut off while I am transferring, here is his direct number." Next he would get our department, and the secretary would ask, "And who may I say is calling?" After that, another screen, and then, "Mr. Guthrie, does Mr. Lee know what this is in reference to?"

Playing this scenario in my mind was all it took for me to tell my secretary to stop screening my calls. "Put all calls straight through to me unless I am unavailable," I told her. I have never had my calls screened since. My wife, Aura, who has been a director of nursing staff development, the director of an LPN school, and director of nurses, has followed the same practice. We didn't phrase it that way in those days, but I now see that Ray Guthrie was simply setting an example of making customer needs (courtesy) more important than his own personal efficiency. And it changed my behavior as well.

THE ACCOUNTING OFFICE CHANGES ITS FOCUS.

Many years ago, at Florida Hospital in Orlando, we had a policy about expense reports that went something like this: Get your report in by the third Friday of the month, and we will get your check back to you within the next week. If you missed the deadline, it might be six weeks before you were reimbursed. This could mean interest charges on your credit card. But that was the policy.

One time I received my check the next day after turning in my expense report. I thought maybe my secretary had invoked a rush order. She said, "No, I didn't do anything. They have a new boss over that area. I think his name is Jim Gravel. Anyway, now the new policy is that if you get your request in by noon, you will get your check the next business day."

Instant turnaround. I have found that it usually takes changing a manager to change the focus of a department from efficiency to service. We are loath to change long-standing policies. We defend them as if our egos were on the line. And who would argue with any manager in healthcare who can show that a policy makes his or her department function more efficiently? Most of the pressure on managers in healthcare today is about costs and efficiency. I have never heard a CEO or vice president say, "Look, I don't care if it is more efficient to do it that way. It just isn't as customer friendly."

I wondered to myself how much efficiency was lost by the new manager who changed the policy to provide 24-hour turnaround on expense reports. Obviously the change did not create more demand. The same number of requests will come in. The same number of checks will have to be cut. And the time it actually takes to cut a check doesn't change. That leaves only the efficiency gained by letting the forms stack up and then going through them all at once, instead of dispatching a few every day or a couple of times a week. Let's say it will now take an extra minute per day of somebody's time. There are 20 working days a month, so for 20 minutes a month, you gain a huge dividend in customer appreciation. Most front line workers would relish the praise they get from these happy customers as well.

IT'S THE MANAGER, NOT THE WORKER.

Recently I visited a hospital near Chicago. I urgently needed the restroom and inquired at the front desk. The receptionist pointed down the hall and explained that the restrooms were in a little alcove off the hallway. I rushed to the alcove and as I rounded the corner, a housekeeper was just backing into the men's room, pulling her cart in with her. I put my hand on her cart and said, "Please hold it just a second. I need to use the restroom."

"I am already in the restroom," she said. "It's temporarily closed.

"You only have one foot in the door," I said, trying to humor her. "Have you been in there yet?" I asked, pointing to the women's room.

"No, but it's always harder to get into the men's restroom, so I have to do it when I get the chance."

"Well, what do you want me to do?" I asked.

"Go to another restroom," she said.

"Where would that be?"

"Downstairs."

"How do I get there?"

"You can either take the elevator or the stairs."

"Which is quicker?"

"I don't know."

"Then I'll take the elevator. Where is that?"

"Down on the other side of the main entrance."

"What floor do I push on the elevator?"

" 'B' for basement."

"When I come off the elevator, which way will I turn?"

"To the right. Then you go to the next hallway and turn right. It will take you by the cafeteria. There are several restrooms there." Then she added, "Sorry."

When I left I thought how it often takes people longer to tell you why they can't do something than it would have taken to just do it in the first place.

I was polite to this housekeeper because I have long since stopped blaming frontline employees for this kind of behavior. She puts efficiency before courtesy because that is what she is taught to do by her manager, who is only interested in how much she gets done in an allotted time and never asks how many people she was friendly to or helped in the process of doing her job. People do not do what their organizations expect. They do what their managers pay attention to.

Not long ago, I was told by someone who had attended one of my seminars that she had gotten excited about the idea of making courtesy more important than efficiency. She told me part of her job entailed entering work orders into the computer. When someone wanted work done, she sent them a sheet of paper to fill out. When the form was filled out, she brought up the same form on the computer and entered in the information. While this might be slightly more efficient, she decided to try bringing the form up on the computer when a person called with a request and to ask the questions in front of her. While they were on the phone, she filled out the work order for them and it was done.

She said, "You know what I discovered? It was actually more efficient in the long run because many times I had to return work orders or call about them because information was often incomplete or incorrect. When I was on the phone with them, these mistakes didn't happen."

I congratulated her on taking the initiative but was taken aback when she went on to tell me that when her manager discovered that she was deviating from the long-established procedure, he put a stop to it. When she tried to show him that it was not taking any longer and it gave better service, his response was, "We are not here to save other people work, we are here to save ourselves work. They can fill out the work orders as they always have."

It has amazed me how many times managers thwart the efforts of frontline employees to institute change, especially if they believe it will compromise some efficiency in the department for the sake of better service. It is as if courtesy is only an afterthought, not a departmental value. Unless courtesy comes ahead of something, it will come ahead of nothing. And no company ever became a great service company with managers who put service and courtesy at the bottom of their priorities.

CAN NURSES MAKE COURTESY MORE IMPORTANT THAN EFFICIENCY?

Several years ago I went in for surgery that required an overnight stay. When I came out from under the general anesthetic, all I wanted to do was sleep. But I had a roommate who was in a great deal of pain. All night long he rang for the nurse on his intercom, and all night long I was awakened by his nurse's voice loudly saying, "Yes, Mr. Jones, what do you need?"

Then he would yell something like, "My leg, could you please come and move my leg?"

It happened at least every hour. I was exhausted by morning and literally hated that wretched intercom. When my wife picked me up in the car and asked how my night had gone, I said, "Awful, just awful."

"Why didn't you tell your nurse?" she asked.

"I'm telling you," I said. "You're a director of nurses. Couldn't you tell your nurses that at night, in semi-private rooms, they might think about slipping quietly into the room instead of waking up the other patient with that loud, annoying intercom? I can see why concern for a patient's privacy is so big in patient satisfaction."

"Now, don't go around the country making an issue about that!" she said. And then I got a lengthy explanation about the ratio of nurses to patients and how you need to know if something the patient wants really needs the nurse or if someone else could do it. By the time she was done, I was convinced that this might be an example of something that can't be changed.

I agreed not to bring it up in my seminars, even though it was such a glaring example of disregard for the patient's privacy (a top driver of satisfaction) and need to sleep. I decided not to talk about it, that is, until I had another experience.

On vacation in Minnesota, I was admitted to United Hospital with a rampant infection and a great deal of pain. They put me in a private room, which delighted me because now if the nurse got called it would be me pushing the button and I would not mind the intercom as I would be in a semi-private room.

I remember how surprised I was when I first pushed the call button and a nurse came into my room quietly and asked me what I needed. After this happened several times, I asked the nurse if the intercom was broken. "No, did you want me to use the intercom?" she asked. Not once in my three-day stay did the nurses ever use the intercom, even though I pressed the call button several times on every shift.

Later I called the director of nurses and told her they should send me one of their patient satisfaction surveys because I would give everybody fives just because the nurses didn't use the intercom.

Her reply was telling. "Well, I guess we just never got into that habit. It's never been part of our nursing culture here to do that." She did add a couple of things that also helped, like no nursing station. They used wall-mounted writing desks by the patient rooms. Also their nurses had cordless phones to take calls directly from physicians and staff. But what impressed me was how they were able to make courtesy more important than efficiency by rarely using the intercom, in spite of the staffing pressures hospitals face today.

INTERNAL SERVICE IS ENTREPRENEURIAL THINKING.

Years ago, when I was vice president at Florida Hospital in Orlando, the head of the marketing and communications department came to my office to have me sign off on a new form they wanted to use with internal departments needing help to produce brochures, advertisements, newsletters, etc. The form asked all the right marketing questions, like: Who is your target audience? What is your key promise? What is the desired action we want the target to take? Do you have this in your budget? How much? What cost center is this going to be charged to? How many printed copies? How many colors? Where and how will it be distributed, aired, or placed? The list went on for two pages. They had thought of everything.

"This will make our jobs much easier," the director said. "Right now, we go to their office and talk it over with them, but that hasn't been very efficient because they often don't know exactly what they want and they haven't given it much thought. This way we will ask them the questions they need to consider. They can think about the answers, and when we get together they will be ready and not waste our time."

As a supportive manager, I thought it was my primary duty to remove barriers and streamline processes so my people could do better work. I used to say to the frontline people, "If you need anything to make your jobs easier, let me know. That's what I'm here for." So of course I signed off on this form.

A couple of months later, the director of one of our internal departments asked me, "Do I have to use the PR department, or can I use an ad agency to produce all the marketing things we need to get our new center of excellence going?"

"Well, you're supposed to use us," I said. "Where would our marketing department be if everybody went outside for the work?"

She didn't seem moved by this logic and pressed her point. "You know, we have a great deal to do, tons of work. And they are so busy. I'm not sure they could handle all we need done."

"In that case they're supposed to decide whether or not to use an outside agency," I said.

"So the answer is I am not allowed to go outside," she said with a touch of exasperation.

"Has something happened in that department that has made you want to go outside?" I asked.

She was reluctant to complain, but I finally got her to tell me how the department had sent her this lengthy form to fill out, which she did. When she had not heard from them in quite a while, she called and asked about her request. They said they had not received it. She went down to the department and showed them where she remembered dropping off the form. After some searching the form turned up on the bottom of an "out" box because the secretary had circled in red the part of the instructions where it clearly stated, "Please type." This was in the days before ordinary departments had computers, and it was a real chore to type on a form using white fluid to cover mistakes.

At the next departmental staff meeting, I decided
few words. The gist of what I said was, "If we had to compe
agencies for every job and this hospital was our major accou
could not afford to lose, would we do anything differently?" From this
question it was not hard to guide the discussion to conclude that we not
only compete on cost and quality, but on service. When the staff said
that an ad agency would probably come to the hospital with a legal pad
of yellow paper and sit down with the client and ask all the questions,
I knew we had come full circle in our thinking. By the end of the
meeting we were ready to scrap something that made our jobs easier
but added work for the clients we served.

There are no sacred departments in a hospital. Any function can be
contracted to other professional agencies that want the business. For a
department director an important question to consider is: *What would
we do differently if we had to compete with outside agencies to keep the
internal clients we have come to take for granted?*

SHIFTING WORK TO OTHER
DEPARTMENTS IS A PHONY EFFICIENCY.

The experience of the marketing questionnaire was all about courtesy
and efficiency. But the insight that struck me was that often the
efficiencies in hospital departments are gained by shifting some of our
work onto another department. When we do this, our department's
efficiency looks better, but from an organizational point of view, this
does not save anything. And if it causes more total work or frustration,
the organization loses—even if one department gains.

Take the example earlier of the department secretary who decided
to take work orders on the phone to provide better service. Her
manager was sure this cost the department in lost efficiency and really
didn't care if it meant more work or inconvenience for the client
department, or customer. But that is a manager with a narrow point of
view that proves to be foolish when examined in its larger context.
When the secretary pointed out that the total time was less because she
didn't have to call back other departments to correct errors anymore,
the manager might have been persuaded just on the issue of efficiency.
But he was so focused on his department's work that he could not bring

himself to consider service in his equation, even if it was more efficient for the hospital overall. It is a phony view of efficiency when it ends up adding to the total cost of doing business for the company, to say nothing of a loss in customer service.

The sad thing is that nobody above this manager will ever know about his discussion with his secretary or the shortsighted decision he made which ends up being less efficient for the organization as a whole. Like so many other budget-minded managers, his shortsightedness and lack of concern for service will actually be rewarded. He is the most likely to be promoted by top management, who will praise him for running an efficient department based on the only numbers they can see–the cost of doing business in that department. No wonder W. Edwards Deming, father of the quality movement, statistician and number–counter extraordinaire, said, "The most important numbers for any organization are unknown and unknowable." Also calling them "invisible figures," this term appears over and over in his seminal book on quality management, *Out of the Crisis*. The value of a happy customer is one of the invisible numbers of supreme importance, but so are the improved efficiency and employee morale from interdepartmental cooperation and process improvement.

By taking the larger view of total process time, adding the department's time and the client's time together, it is surprising how often doing it the way the customer wishes ends up being the most cost-effective way to do the job, even if the results do not show up in visible numbers. If it is also less frustrating for the customer, then there is a double win—a win in overall efficiency and a win in customer satisfaction.

ONE SIMPLE RULE ALIGNS EVERYTHING.

Deming listed 14 points that form the roadmap to corporate excellence and quality. Number 9 is "breaking down the barriers between departments." At any leadership workshop where I have had groups make a list of barriers to service excellence, there are two that I can predict will always come up–lack of communication between departments, and lack of cross functional teamwork. The desire to create a management culture characterized by teamwork is so pervasive that hospitals spend considerable sums conducting team-building retreats. The most rigorous retreats involve physical activities, which demand teamwork to succeed. Another popular variation is to play games based on hypothetical situations where it takes teamwork to succeed.

In spite of a huge cottage industry that has arisen to provide such team-building retreats, I have yet to find one group that feels any improvement in teamwork between departments ever resulted even in the first few months from the retreat. They had fun. They got to know people's personality better. They became more comfortable with people they did not know before. They saw their administrator and vice presidents in a new light. They had a wonderful time playing together. They would rather have had the retreat than not. But as for any work-related improvements, the results were nil. When people return to the same environment, with the same management structures in place, the same attitudes and behaviors will not change as a result of getting better acquainted with people in a different setting.

Accountabilities drive structure and structure drives culture. Because this concept is so fundamental and powerful, let me repeat that. *Accountabilities drive structure and structure drives culture.* Any leader who is striving to change the culture of a hospital would do well to ponder this key principle: You can't change the fruits of a tree without changing the roots. In chapter 5 of this book, I address this more in depth, but here is where I want to indicate how powerful Disney's simple principle of making courtesy more important than efficiency is. It strikes at a cultural root. Do you have a tree rooted in structures that support this rule, or do you have a tree rooted in structures that support primarily the fruits of unit efficiency?

But now we come to a surprising paradox: by putting courtesy and service first, our problem with phony efficiency virtually disappears. So do problems with communication and teamwork between departments. One rule, if followed by all departments, aligns the entire culture. Talk about an elegant model! This means that we can actually get the fruits of overall corporate efficiency when we subordinate departmental efficiency for the sake of courtesy and responsiveness (the most important aspects of service). Figure 2.1 demonstrates the line of thinking behind this paradox.

Figure 2.1: The Efficiency/Courtesy Paradox

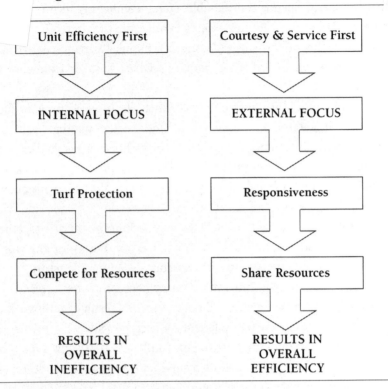

Unit Efficiency First	Courtesy & Service First
INTERNAL FOCUS	EXTERNAL FOCUS
Turf Protection	Responsiveness
Compete for Resources	Share Resources
RESULTS IN OVERALL INEFFICIENCY	RESULTS IN OVERALL EFFICIENCY

The ultimate shortcut to getting the best overall efficiency is to focus on service and make it more important than efficiency. As long as department directors have to answer only for their own labor costs, cross-functional savings and teamwork are not likely to happen. And the waste will go unmeasured and unnoticed as it gets invisibly absorbed by the organization. Place service above efficiency, however, and the internal customer will speak up and document the waste caused by poor service delivery. Working together as internal service provider and customer department, these inefficiencies would be identified and addressed in a culture of teamwork and responsiveness instead of competition. Again, this one rule can change the entire management culture more dramatically than twenty team-building retreats. What top management needs to figure out is how to foster a climate in which departments and their managers are held accountable and rewarded for service instead of being punished for it, as they would be under conventional hospital budget monitoring and accountability systems.

IS THERE A LIMIT TO HOW FAR
YOU CAN GO WITH THIS PRINCIPLE?

That's a good question. Certainly my wife felt it would be asking too much to expect overworked nurses to stop using their intercoms to respond to patient calls–until she discovered a hospital where the nurses are doing that. Often the limits are in our own minds and based on the way we have always thought were our constraints.

A couple of years ago at Avista Hospital in Louisville, Colorado, I was doing a series of 75-minute talks to front line staff as they rotated through all day. During the break I would step out into the hallway or go to the restroom. After a while I noticed that I had greeted the same food service worker several times pushing a fresh food cart. Since it was often between meals, I wondered if he was late or early. When I said something to him about it, he grinned and said, "We deliver food all day long because we have room service here for anybody who wants it any time of the day."

"For just patients, or their families, too?" I asked.

"Oh, no. Anybody. Families too. Even nurses can order room service to where they are working."

"Nurses too?" I said incredulously.

"Not only that, we also deliver to the staff in our doctors' offices!"

"How can you do that?"

"It's easy. The doctors' offices are in a building attached to the hospital. In fact, I just go down this hallway and I'm there."

Later, when I had the chance, I talked on the phone with Doug McCaw, the director of food service. The first question out of my mouth was, "How can you afford to do this?"

His answer was a stunning example of what can happen in a culture based on making courtesy more important than efficiency, and the truth behind the amazing paradox illustrated in Figure 2.1.

"Do you know our CEO, John Sackett?" he asked.

"Yes," I said.

"Then you know what a fanatic he is about great service. We had the idea that if our department really wanted to give great service, we would be offering room service any time during the day, just like a hotel. John said, 'Go for it, and let's see what happens.' So I did.

"And it didn't break the bank?" I asked.

"No, not at all. We found it actually saved money. In no time we were serving twice as many meals."

"Didn't the labor costs go through the roof?"

"Well, not really. We saved money on a per meal basis. Also, we cut way down on waste because people were getting only what they ordered and eating when they wanted to instead of throwing the food away. What we saved on volume and waste paid for the labor, so it turned out to be a wash. Then we went to John and told him that since this has gone so well, why not make room service available for the nurses too. And again he said, 'Go for it.' And we did. Next thing we knew we had tripled our volume with even lower cost per meal. So we decided to open it up for the doctors' offices too. Now we serve the same number of meals as a hospital quadruple our size. But I could never have done it without a CEO like John who encourages us to try things in the name of great service."

Later, in a conversation with John Sackett, the CEO, I learned that the entire community of Louisville has heard about the room service anybody can get at Avista Hospital. Even the doctors rave about it. When an independent research company was doing market research in the area, they discovered a level of loyalty from physicians and the community to Avista Hospital that far exceeded any hospital they had ever encountered in their research. Asked about such high raves, the typical telephone response was, "Did you know, they provide room service to patients and their families and even their employees?" Here was loyalty generated throughout a community where the word of mouth was most often praise for the food service.

So, how far can you go down the road of making courtesy more important than efficiency? Probably lots farther than most managers believe.

CHAPTER 3 REGARD PATIENT SATISFACTION AS FOOL'S GOLD

In the 1980s we developed our own patient-satisfaction survey at Florida Hospital, using a five-point scale for each question. We asked patients to grade us according to:

A = Excellent
B = Good
C = Satisfactory
D = Poor
F = Failure

To us everything above a "D" meant the customer was satisfied. Typically the percentage of satisfied patients was in the high 80s. What we showed our employees was a numerical average, or a GPA–like 3.4 or 2.8–on each question, by nursing unit.

Over the years of using this scale, it became apparent that a number like 3.1 meant little or nothing to a frontline employee. There was nothing about the numbers that motivated anyone or caused alarm if the number went down the next quarter. Only a few managers paid any attention to them at all, and top management was focused on other indicators so didn't make an issue of the patient-satisfaction scores.

Besides, we had no idea how we compared with other hospitals because we did not share a database with other facilities using the same questions in the same way.

After a few years of crunching our own numbers, we hired a company to do the work for us. This way we had the advantage of a comparative database and could see how Florida Hospital numbers stacked up with others. Top management appreciated the ability to compare, and as long as we were in the top quartile, little else was done with the survey results. The average employee still found the numbers meaningless in terms of how to do his or her job better, and managers put the data on a shelf.

Now that I have seen the survey instruments and patient-satisfaction scores from many hospitals, I suspect that not one hospital in 20 uses its patient-satisfaction scores to improve performance. I also suspect that not one in a hundred hospital employees has any idea what the patient-satisfaction scores are from quarter to quarter.

DISNEY DOES NOT MEASURE GUEST SATISFACTION.

When I went to work at Disney, I was anxious to see their customer-satisfaction data. I was certain their scores would be far higher than those of a typical hospital. After all, how hard is it to please a family at a fancy resort, on vacation, being entertained all day? Compare Disney customers to hospital patients, and they are at opposite ends on a scale of difficulty. Hospital employees have a much tougher customer to please, and a much tougher job to do. The hospital experience cannot be standardized like a ride at Disney. Their employees spend a few minutes interacting with their guests; we spend hours, even days and weeks. Comparing our "moments of truth" with theirs had to be like comparing real mice with Mickey Mouse. We were in the real world of pain and suffering and grief. They were in the land of fantasy, pixie dust, and family fun. Could any two organizations be more different? One day I had the opportunity to see what kind of guest satisfaction scores they got at Disney and compare them to ours in the health care business.

When I became a cast member at Disney, I wore an oval badge with my first name, FRED, in large letters. This badge allowed me to go backstage into areas not open to guests. On one of my very first scouting trips, I went backstage at one of Disney's luxury family resorts. On a large wall near the cast dining room was a gigantic poster that listed seven or eight questions that determine guest satisfaction at the resort. Beside each question was a percentage number. I assumed this number represented the percentage of guests that had indicated they were satisfied with the resort's performance on that item on a questionnaire.

What surprised me was how *low* these scores were compared to the scores we generally see in hospitals. The highest score was somewhere in the high 70s, while the lowest score was in the 60s. Typically in a hospital scores run 10 to 20 percentage points higher than that! Given my perceptions about how much easier it must be to deliver guest satisfaction at Disney than in a hospital, I was surprised, almost shocked.

I thought I must be missing something, so I stopped a person who looked like a manager and asked, "Are those the questions you ask your guests?"

"Yes."

"I'm surprised at the percentages," I continued. "Is that the percentage of respondents who say they are satisfied with your performance on that item?"

"Not exactly," the person replied. "That is the percentage of respondents who said they are very satisfied. We use a five-point scale. A four means you are satisfied. A five means you are very satisfied."

"Oh," I said. "I came from a hospital where we combined the threes, fours, and fives because they are all satisfied."

The person chuckled. "If we did that, all our scores would probably be 99 or 100 percent, and what would that tell our employees? That we are perfect? But we are not perfect unless everyone gives us fives."

Later I spoke to my boss at Disney about this encounter. He gave me an article from the *Harvard Business Review* on customer loyalty. In it, the authors presented research showing that satisfied customers are not necessarily loyal. On a scale of one to five, a customer who marks a four is six times more likely to defect than a customer who marks a five. In other words, there is a six-fold increase in customer loyalty between fours and fives. Disney does not display guest-satisfaction scores to its cast members; it shows them only the percentage of respondents giving fives to the questions. They are not measuring customer satisfaction; they are measuring customer *loyalty*. And when you think about it, customer loyalty, not mere satisfaction, is the only protection any organization has against serious competition in its future. Security, then, is not rooted in patient satisfaction, it is linked to their loyalty.

PATIENT SATISFACTION IS FOOL'S GOLD.

After spending years touting patient satisfaction, it was unsettling to learn that patient satisfaction is fool's gold. It looks valuable but you can't take it to the bank if it doesn't mean that patients will be loyal and sing your praises.

When I analyze my own evaluation process, I readily understand the difference between satisfaction and loyalty. Let's say I receive a survey in the mail from a place I had stayed for several days. I think back over my experience and I remember nothing special and nothing bad. Everyone did exactly as I expected. Everyone was polite. Everything worked. My room was clean. Nothing stood out one way or the other. What would I put on the survey? Probably a four–satisfied. When you can't remember anything, you are satisfied. It takes something memorable to turn an ordinary, satisfactory experience into something special. Either something happened that you remember as bad, or something happened that you remember as special. Dissatisfaction comes from the bad. Loyalty is generated by memorable things that happen that we didn't expect.

One of my client hospitals is in Knoxville, Tennessee. The hotel I had used on my first visit was full, so I stayed at the Residence Inn on my second trip. In the middle of the week of my stay I was walking to my car one morning and could see from a distance that someone had left a note on my windshield. My first thought was that I must have done something wrong or that someone had scratched my car. It was a business card. On the card were these handwritten words: "Have a good day. Windows on us! Maintenance Department." I looked down the line of cars, and, sure enough, every one had a note.

In all my travels I have never heard of hotel staff ⊂
guests' windshields. It was a surprise. In one stroke an e₁
created customer loyalty from a jaded traveler. Because of ↻
on only one morning of my stay, the Residence Inn got my   ..ued
loyalty and became my first choice in many other cities as well.

I wondered how an organization gets its employees to do special
things that are not in their job descriptions. When I returned to the
hotel that evening, I asked for an appointment to visit with the general
manager. Her name was Debra Stacey. I showed her the card that I
found on my windshield and said, "How do you get your employees to
do this kind of thing? Is this your idea or his?"

She looked at the card and smiled. "No, it's his idea. But we have a
saying around here that goes 'If we don't do something special for our
guests, they won't remember us. And if they don't remember us, why
would they come again?' "

LOYALTY IS HARD TO GET, BUT NOT AS HARD AS YOU WOULD THINK.

It can be discouraging to know that after doing everything to
perfection, after meeting all our standards of performance and courtesy,
we still have not created a loyal customer, merely a satisfied customer.
That makes it seem as though loyalty is nearly impossible to attain. But
in my experience, though it takes somebody doing something special
beyond what is expected, it doesn't take everybody doing something
special all the time. It takes only one brief experience on only one day
of a stay. Just so, it takes only one brief comment or moment of
rudeness to ruin an otherwise perfect stay. It's this *law of the memorable
event* that determines dissatisfaction and loyalty.

One washed windshield on only one day earned the loyalty of a
frequent traveler who spends thousands of dollars a year on hotels. And
that one event changed my ratings on any survey from the Residence
Inn from four to five (except in their case, the company that does
Marriott surveys uses a scale from one to ten). One inappropriate
remark can ruin a stay. One effort beyond a person's job description can
win the same customer's loyalty. It's just that so few employees ⌐
beyond their task to create loyalty.

Debra Stacey invited me to attend one of her staff meetings. I asked when the next one would be. She said they had a full staff meeting at 10 A.M. every day in the lobby. Any guest can listen in. That surprised me. The next day I went. First they dispatched with any birthdays. Then Debra asked if anyone was needing special prayers on their behalf. There was an announcement about a sorority booking most of the rooms for the weekend. "They are probably thinking that we have bellmen here, which of course we don't. But it would be a big help if everyone would be available to give them a hand with their bags, just the same." Then they brainstormed some potential problems that might arise from such a large slumber party and talked about how to handle difficult situations.

Before adjourning the meeting, Debra asked if anybody had done something special for a guest. Cindy, the receptionist, said that a man had called down the day before to see if he could get a needle and thread. She had asked him why he needed it and when he said it was to sew on a button, she offered to sew it on for him, which pleased him very much.

What I saw was a manager's style of leadership. Daily huddles. Taking a personal interest in each employee. Making the guest's stay memorable. Talking about personal things in every staff meeting. Praising and role-modeling employees that go the extra mile to make sure the guest will remember something special about his or her stay. Creating loyalty, one person at a time. It was no surprise to me when she later confided, "We have the highest ratings of any Marriott property in our category."

WHEN CUSTOMERS ARE SATISFIED, THERE ARE NO STORIES.

Sometimes I will ask people to tell about a place that has captured their loyalty. Every time there is a story. Or I might ask about a place that has lost their loyalty and where they would never return. Again, there is

. What seems to be a major component of both loyalty
ction are stories. A satisfied person has no story to tell.
nt just as expected. It is the unexpected event that makes

a stay memorable. For every loyal customer, there is usually a special story.

I like Chinese food. My parents were missionaries to China, where I grew up. Chinese food was home cooking for me. When I first moved to Orlando, I tried a different Chinese restaurant every week. My requirements were that they cook in the spicy Szechuan style my mother preferred and speak Mandarin to me. This was my only chance to practice the language that was fading in my memory. If they did these two things in a courteous way and made over my ability to speak their language, I was satisfied. I kept trying new restaurants, not because I wasn't satisfied but because I was curious. It meant more variety and more Chinese people to meet.

I happened to return to one of the restaurants, the Orient IV, after several weeks, and the owner remembered me by name. During the meal he came over to our table and carried on a lengthy conversation in Chinese with me. He asked me if I especially liked any particular dish when growing up in China. I told him about a dish our family cook used to make in Taiwan. It had three ingredients: *dofu-gan* (an especially firm, savory tofu), *tsa-tsai* (a pickled vegetable from central China), and bell peppers. He laughed and said he had hoped to make the dish for me but he didn't know where he could get the very rare (for those days) *dofu-gan* and the pickled vegetable. I told him that in all my travels in America I had not found that style of tofu either. It's too bad, really, because Americans think the only kind of tofu is the white, tasteless variety that is familiar here. Actually there are as many kinds of tofu in China as there are cheeses in America.

A month or two later I returned to the Orient IV where I had had the conversation about my favorite dish, and the manager exclaimed, "Where have you been? We have been watching for you. I have found the things to make your special food. When you left last time, I asked my cook if he knew where to find the dofu-gan. He said he knew a family in Miami who made it. We called them and they sent it right away. It is in my freezer. We also got a can of the tsa-tsai. Now I can make your favorite dish. Tell me how to make it, and I will make it for you."

And so that night I had a dish I had not tasted since I was a boy. You can imagine what happened to my loyalty. Instead of Chinese food once a week, I was now going several times a week to the same restaurant and bringing all my friends. Why? Because I had a story to tell. A story about someone going out of his way to please a guest.

Is it hard? Yes, but not as hard as one might think. It takes just one person, during one visit, becoming personally involved by doing something special. The owner even put the dish on his menu when he had new ones printed up, and called it the Fred Lee Special. I once asked him if anybody ever ordered the Fred Lee Special, and he said, "Yes. Many times. They think Fred Lee is me!"

MOST METHODS USED TO KEEP CUSTOMERS WON'T WORK FOR HOSPITALS.

Most businesses have a simple measurement for loyalty—the percentage of customers who return for repeat purchases. Since getting customers to come back is the main goal, there are a number of practices available to businesses to get customers to return that are not open to hospitals, such as:

Better prices
Convenient location
Frequent-buyer perks
Special discounts and sales
Superior brand recognition

All of these are popular ways to get customers to return, but none is useful for hospitals. An airline can keep my business with frequent-flyer miles, but can you imagine a hospital receptionist saying, "Mr. Lee, I see this is your ninth visit to our hospital. Did you know your next visit will be free?" Neither can we create demand for surgeries by offering two-for-one specials. People don't go to a hospital because it's more convenient, either. They will drive much farther for what they perceive to be a better facility.

Unlike other service companies then, hospitals have only one way to create loyalty—the patient's personal experience. And they have only one way to measure loyalty–by what the patient says about their visit. That's why surveys of patient perceptions are so important for hospitals. It is through surveys that we find out what percentage of patients are singing our praises.

If the only real source of loyalty for hospitals is the patient's experience, and the only test of that experience is what patients say about it, learning what creates the best experience for a patient should be our primary goal. After the first edition of *The Loyalty Effect* became a business book best-seller, its author, Frederick F. Richheld, was astonished at how quickly business leaders rushed to develop customer retention programs. He wrote in the preface to his paperback edition:

> Rather than investing in the creation of mutually beneficial partnerships founded on the principles of loyalty, executives experimented with shortcuts such as frequent flier miles and jackpot schemes. They presumed that their marketing departments could manipulate their way to customer loyalty. "Customer relationship management" tools became the rage, as if one could manage (and manipulate) a partner into being loyal. The truth is that loyalty must be earned…[1]

In the case of hospitals, there is no other choice.

FOR PATIENTS, LOYALTY COMES FROM COMPASSION.

Recently I asked my wife to bring home from work a stack of unsolicited comments from patients who had stayed at her hospital to see what words patients used in describing the behaviors that made them love the staff at the hospital. I decided that the ones raving about their care, especially since they were completely spontaneous, represented loyalty. Typical were comments like these:

"All the staff were terrific (and very shorthanded and overworked). Julia is to be especially commended for her kindness and compassion."

"My daughter received excellent care and concern from Judy (fourth-floor nursing)."

"I wish to thank the nurse Herma who was so thoughtful and considerate while taking care of my mother."

"I have to let you know that you have above excellent, caring, professional, loving, understanding nurses on or in your staff team. I'm sure the charge nurse or supervisor of this floor has something to do with how these good people treat us, keep up the good work. We will definitely refer anyone to this peds department."

I decided to underline the adjectives used in these patient comments and make a list of them. Those used most often, I thought, might indicate the kind of qualities that create loyalty. Below is the list of adjectives that were used at least once. The number of additional times the same adjective was mentioned is noted after each word:

If one picks out the synonyms for compassion (the words most repeated) there is an amazing consistency in the qualities that have the greatest impact on patient loyalty. They comprise at least two-thirds of all the adjectives used. Courtesy synonyms comprise a distant second place. Competence synonyms are the least mentioned. This is not because courtesy and competence are unimportant. It's because they are expected, but doing what is expected does not earn unsolicited raves.

Caring, cares, cared +32	Knowledgeable +2
Kind, kindness +24	Thoughtful +2
Compassionate +15	Bedside manner +2
Help, helpfulness +15	Takes time +1
Comfort, comforting +13	Courteous
Concerned +6	Gentle
Listens +4	Nice
Loving +3	Committed
Understanding +2	Cheerful
Empathy +2	Informative
Tender +1	Warm
Sensitive	Upbeat
Reassuring	Generous
Selfless	Softness
	Pleasant
Friendly +8	Supportive
Professional +9	Quick +3
Attention, attentive +7	Proficient
Sweet +3	Prompt
Respect +3	Hardworking, efficient
Polite +3	Conscientious
Patient +3	Competent
Smiling +2	

Loyalty is gained by showing more than simple c⟨...⟩ cases, it comes from being engaged with the patient in ⟨...⟩ compassion.

In my conversations with patients the same is ⟨...⟩ stories of loyalty that I hear have something to do with compassion. ⟨...⟩ might illustrate the link between staff performance and patient evaluations in the following way:

There are three levels of caring—competence, courtesy, and compassion.

Figure 3.1: Three Levels of Caring

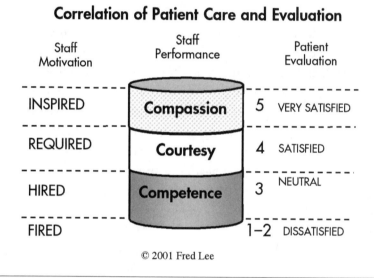

Correlation of Patient Care and Evaluation

Staff Motivation	Staff Performance	Patient Evaluation	
INSPIRED	Compassion	5	VERY SATISFIED
REQUIRED	Courtesy	4	SATISFIED
HIRED	Competence	3	NEUTRAL
FIRED		1–2	DISSATISFIED

© 2001 Fred Lee

The first level of care is competence. We hire healthcare personnel for their competence. We continually develop their competence on the job as they learn to use new equipment and adapt to new protocols in medicine. Competence is the level at which clinical staff is hired and fired.

Our next level of care is courtesy. Courtesy is not usually in our criteria for hiring, but if the organization begins to focus on customer needs and wants, courtesy quickly becomes something that is required. We stress it in orientation. We call it service excellence. We write scripts to standardize courteous behaviors. These behaviors become part of our

scriptions and performance reviews. We might not fire anybody
, lacks skills in courtesy, as we would with clinical incompetencies,
ut we do try to make it something that is required. And repeated
examples of outright rudeness can be grounds for dismissal.

Finally there is the emotional level of caring. It is clearly beyond
ordinary courtesy. Let's call it compassion. It is not something we hire
for. It is not something that can be required. We don't fire people who
don't know how to express it. It appears to be an action that springs
spontaneously from a person who is "inspired."

Patients expect a certain basic competence from everyone in
healthcare. When nurses or therapists do their jobs, it's doing what they
get paid to do. When we do our job without much warmth, we may
think we are doing what we are hired to do, but that is worth about a
three (neutral or good) on a patient-satisfaction survey. If we do our job
with warmth and courtesy, the patient will probably raise that three to
a *four* (satisfied or very good). But notice that we are still in the range
of meeting patient expectations. To exceed the patient's expectations
and get a *five* (very satisfied or excellent), it takes somebody who goes
beyond doing a task in a courteous way. Because of the emotional
distress that accompanies most healthcare problems, this usually means
doing or saying something that shows a genuine concern for the
patient's state of mind. It means exhibiting some heartfelt empathy for
the patient's anxiety and pain.

Judy, a good friend of mine, told me a personal story that provides
an example of what I mean. Her life took a shattering turn when her
physician told her she had breast cancer and needed a radical
mastectomy. She said the news was so devastating that she was nearly
immobilized by fear and anxiety. She shed many tears and wondered
how this would affect her life and her marriage. Her troubled thoughts
were so intrusive that she often found it difficult even to listen to a
person speaking to her.

On the night after her surgery Judy recalled holding her emotions
together for the sake of her husband while he sat by her bed. Late that
night he finally turned off the light above her bed and went home to get
some needed rest. After he left, a feeling of loneliness and grief engulfed
her; the reservoir of tears broke and she began to cry softly to herself.

Judy's nurse came into her room with a little tray in her hand. She turned on the light above her bed, and when she saw Judy crying, she turned off the light and put down the tray she was holding. The nurse then pulled up a chair and took Judy's hand in her own and held it for a long time without saying a word. "It was like an angel had entered my room," Judy said. "When I was all done crying, I thanked the nurse and told her I was OK. Only then did the nurse stand up and say something. 'I have brought you something to sleep,' she said. I will never forget what that nurse did as long as I live."

When I asked Judy how the rest of her stay went, she recalled several things that did not go very well, but that nurse became the symbol of her hospitalization. She expressed loyalty to that hospital because of the compassionate behavior of one nurse on one shift on just one critical day of pain.

What Judy's nurse did cannot be something that is required. It was especially meaningful to the patient because it was spontaneous. It was the tender connection between two people, one in great emotional pain, the other willing to enter the patient's world for a few minutes and experience that pain through empathy. Sometimes words are unnecessary. Most of us would call what happened to Judy an example of compassion, something the nurse did because she felt *inspired* to do it.

COMPASSION ALSO CREATES LOYALTY TO PHYSICIANS.

During my research for a presentation to physicians, entitled *Understanding Patient Loyalty and the Predisposition to Sue*, I came across numerous studies that showed a strong relationship between physician communication and malpractice lawsuits. In fact, nearly three-quarters of the lawsuits against physicians can be classified as minor, temporary, or emotional. In other words, somebody became angry about something other than clinical outcomes.

The most ambitious study I read about was reported in the February 1997 issue of *The Journal of the American Medical Association*. The physicians studied came from two segments: frequently–sued physicians and never-sued physicians. The researchers made 1,250 audiotapes of physician-patient conversations. Through double-blind methods they analyzed every sentence uttered by the physician and sorted all these statements into 38 specific categories under three major headings:

Content	(information gathering, assessment, diagnosis)
Process	(orientation, explaining, preparing what to expect, patient flow)
Emotional	(validating, empathizing, warmth, humor, dealing with worries)

In the first category, which I would call the "competence" level, there was no significant difference between those frequently sued and those never sued. Clinical practice was the same in both groups. There was some minor difference in the second category, but the most significant was in the last category–emotional–which fit perfectly with our labeling of "compassion."

After one of my seminars, a participant told me that I might be interested in why she had changed family practice doctors.

"It seemed rather trivial at the time, so I didn't tell my previous doctor the real reason I asked to have my children's charts forwarded to a new doctor," she said. "My little boy—he's about five—had a bad sore throat, but our regular doctor was on vacation when I called for an appointment. The receptionist told me it would be impossible to be seen that day, so I called around to find someone who could see us right away. We got right in to another place and met this new doctor. I'll never forget this simple little thing he did. When he asked my child to open his mouth and say 'ah,' he looked inside and said, in the kindest tone, 'My goodness! I can see how sore your throat is. That really hurts, doesn't it?' When he took a culture with a bit of cotton on a stick, he said, 'We're going to see what kind of germ is hurting you, and then we are going to give you the right medicine to kill them all!' Then he turned to me and said, 'I think he has strep throat.' "

I asked her how that was different from what her regular doctor would have done. She said, "My regular doctor is very professional and polite–don't get me wrong–but he would have simply looked down my son's throat and taken the culture without saying anything except maybe, 'Say "ah" for me.' And 'This won't hurt.' Then he would have told me it might be strep throat."

This story is a perfect illustration of the premise that satisfied patients are not necessarily loyal and that compassion is often the deciding factor in patient loyalty.

FAMILY MEMBERS NEED EMPATHY TOO.

On one of my trips, I received an urgent call that my mother had been in a terrible automobile accident, in which she had fallen asleep at the wheel and hit a tree. In the accident my father was killed and my mother had broken her neck, her sternum, one leg in three places, and the other leg just above the knee. My sister, who called, didn't think our 84-year-old mother would make it through the extensive surgery required. The hospital that originally received her in the emergency department decided that her condition was beyond their surgical skills, and she was taken by helicopter to the University of California Davis Medical Center in Sacramento.

I took the first plane I could get to be at her side. On the plane I remember thinking about her coming out of surgery and my getting there shortly after she had arrived in ICU. I wondered if the nurses in ICU would be strict about how long I could spend with my mother. I pictured them telling me that I could spend only 10 minutes out of the hour with her. The more I thought about being chased out of ICU, the more I decided I was going to be belligerent about my rights to be with my mother as long as she wanted me there. I even thought about saying in my most assertive tone, "You guys are in the dark ages with a policy like this. My wife is a director of nursing at a hospital with unlimited ICU visitation. All the studies done in recent years show that patients who have a loved one by the bed night and day have better outcomes than patients who don't."

I finally arrived at the ICU waiting room, pushed the button on the intercom, and told them who I was and who I had come to visit. As I walked into the unit, I was a time-bomb ready to go off if anybody tried to limit my time with my mother. When I entered her room, it was a shock to see her on a ventilator. Her head was in a steel halo with rods running from the rim into her skull. Her face was swollen beyond recognition. Her bandages made her seem twice as big in the bed.

Off to one side of her bed was her nurse facing a bank of electronic equipment with blinking lights. She was writing on my mother's chart. I hoped she didn't notice me enter the room as I went over to the other side of the bed and took my mother's hand. Not knowing if she was awake or not, I said softly, "Mother, this is Fred and I am here now to be with you." I felt a gentle squeeze and knew she heard and understood me.

As if on cue, the nurse turned and looked at me. I thought, *Here it comes. Give it your best shot, lady.* But instead, the nurse smiled and said, "My, my, my, you should see what your touch just did to your mother's vital signs. It's amazing. We need you here all the time!"

We need you here all the time! Could she have come up with a more perfectly timed thing to say? It was as if she had read my mind and in one gracious comment had made me feel needed and welcome, an essential part of the healing team. That's what I mean by something beyond courtesy, something that shows awareness and compassion. To be prepared to say the perfect thing, she had to be aware of my presence, its effect on the monitors, my mother's high level of anxiety, and how much I needed the reassurance that I was not an intrusion on her work or the patient's well-being. It was one of the memorable moments I had during those weeks I spent helping my mother recuperate and return to full health again.

ASKING THE RIGHT QUESTIONS IS THE KEY TO REVEALING THE LOYALTY FACTOR.

After years of studying the patient-satisfaction surveys from the industry's major providers and many self-surveys done by hospitals and regional systems, I have discovered that a shocking number of hospitals are not asking the questions that have the highest correlation with patient loyalty. This means that their patient-satisfaction surveys have a serious blind spot. Most administrators who put great stock in surveys believe that the most important questions are being asked. This may not be true. What matters most in creating loyalty is still an influence, even if we do not ask about it. If we do not ask about it, concentrating harder on the questions that merely do what is expected may improve the percentage of satisfaction but completely miss what creates loyalty.

Through the years, the Press Ganey and the Gallup surveys that include questions with "care," "compassion," or "concern" in them have the highest correlation with overall satisfaction and loyalty, typically over a .64 coefficient of correlation. The trouble with many other survey companies is that they do not ask these questions at all. It's no wonder. When surveys are first circulated through nursing for approval, the nursing staff often see these questions as too subjective and not behavior specific. They say, "How can you require compassion? How can you evaluate it?" Consequently, questions like these get scratched from the survey. Unfortunately, the patient knows what compassion looks, sounds, or feels like and responds to it whether we want it as a question or not.

The CEO of a hospital that uses the Gallup survey once showed me two scatter diagrams with numbered dots placed on an axis. Each dot represented a question on their patient-satisfaction survey. A shift toward the upper right quadrant was a shift in the desired direction for improvement. The two charts were from two different quarters. What puzzled the CEO was the fact that one could clearly see that nearly all the dots had shifted toward the upper right quadrant in the second, most recent chart, but on the question "Overall how satisfied were you with your stay?" the score had gone down.

"How can it be that the individual responses showed a major improvement, but the overall satisfaction went down?" he asked.

I looked at the dots with the tiny numbers beside them. Two of the dots were almost on top of each other and caught my eye. The whole cluster of dots had indeed clearly moved in the right direction, but these two dots, on close inspection, had actually gone in the opposite direction. "What are these two responses?" I asked.

He looked them up in the key and said, "One is 'Nurses showed care and compassion,' and the other is 'Staff anticipated your needs.'" The very two questions that Gallup had identified as having the highest correlation with overall satisfaction and loyalty were the two questions that appeared to dramatically influence overall satisfaction.

Here was a statistically generated graphic showing how it is possible to improve systems, improve the registration process, improve explaining tests and procedures, improve waits, and improve the performance of ancillary and support services in the patient's eyes; yet all of these combined improvements could not raise overall satisfaction when staff miss the opportunities to anticipate people's needs and show some empathy in their times of stress, pain, and grief.

Unless patient satisfaction surveys have a question or two about compassion, caring, comfort or empathy, they are avoiding the most important questions that correlate with overall satisfaction and certainly loyalty. Without such questions we run the risk of creating a blind spot in our survey process and consequently may miss the most potent influence on high scores.

---

1. Frederick F. Reichheld, *The Loyalty Effect: The Hidden Force Behind Growth, Profits and Lasting Value,* (Boston: Harvard Business School Press, 2001), p x.

CHAPTER

MEASURE TO IMPROVE, NOT TO IMPRESS

Let's imagine checking into a Disney resort hotel. Pretend that at the registration desk they show you a copy of their guest satisfaction survey and let you know how important this survey is to them. They explain that they want you to be able to put a *five* (very satisfied) for each question. And then they say, "If, at any time, you do not think we have earned a *five*, please call us and let us know so we can rectify the situation immediately."

Let's also pretend that after a couple of days at the resort you get a knock at the door. It is the general manager of the hotel. He asks if he can come in and talk about something with you. Once more you are told, now by a person in authority, that this survey means a lot to Disney, and if, for any reason, you do not think you can conscientiously give a *five* to every question, you are expected to call the general manager and let him know.

You check out on Sunday morning. At the front desk let's imagine you are confronted a third time with the guest survey and told that it will be arriving in the mail for you to fill out and return to the company that is doing the surveys for Disney. Is there any reason you cannot give a five on every question you are asked, because if there is, it is only fair that Disney know about it right away and have a chance to address it with their staff.

What would you think if this really happened at a Disney resort? A little too eager to influence your response? Pressuring you? Intimidation? Pushy? Yet hospitals all over the country are doing just that. Why? I believe it's because hospitals have joined healthcare systems where many hospitals compete to have the best numbers in the system and bonuses are tied to their rankings. This makes it more important to managers to get high scores than to get honest feedback.

PRESSURING CUSTOMERS IS AN OUTGROWTH OF COMPETITIVE COMPENSATION.

As far as I know, pressuring guests to give a higher than intended satisfaction score on a survey is not being done in hotels. So if hotels don't do it, where are we getting this practice? Through personal experience I know of at least one other industry in which competition, and corresponding financial remuneration, has caused managers to try to look better than they are by getting customers to overstate their actual assessment.

I ran into this recently when I took my car to a dealer for some repairs. Stapled to my bill was a form letter from the service manager. (See Figure 4.1.) Notice the blatant attempt to get me to turn a five-point scale into a two-point scale, "satisfied" or "not satisfied." This manager is obviously not interested in the difference between a satisfied and a loyal customer. He is going to considerable lengths to get me to eliminate all but the highest score. Observe how the row of boxes representing the top of the scale (Excellent) is separated from the rest by a line all the way down the list. At the top of the column, just to emphasize how undesirable it is for me to give anything less than the highest rating, there is a word that screams out at the reader: the word "Failing." In other words a 4 (satisfied) means they failed! I would think a 1 (very dissatisfied) is the score that means they failed. But this service manager is trying to get me to give his service department a five (very satisfied) just in case I was thinking a 3 or a 4 (satisfied) might do.

Figure 4.1: Service-rating Form

I know you had a choice of where to service your vehicle and I would like to thank you for the opportunity to earn your business. I also know that if I expect to build a strong customer base, I need to make sure that you are completely satisfied with your service experience here today.

Below is a list of questions that may appear on a questionaire from my dealership or possibly even Honda. Although some of them seem to rate our entire operation, in fact they all rate my personal performance and the scores become part of my permanent record. If you feel I have not earned all *"Excellent"* or *"Yes"* ratings, please call and allow me the opportunity to correct any of my failures or shortcomings. While my score is very important, any desire to earn and keep your business is far more important. If there is any situation where I may be of assistance now or in the future, please let me know.

EXCELLENT   FAILING

	EXCELLENT		FAILING		
Promptness and courtesy in greeting and writing your order	☐	☐	☐	☐	☐
Service advisors knowledge and expertise	☐	☐	☐	☐	☐
Treated in an honest and straightforward manner	☐	☐	☐	☐	☐
Amount of time spent with you	☐	☐	☐	☐	☐
Understanding your service or repair request	☐	☐	☐	☐	☐
Length of time to complete this service or repair	☐	☐	☐	☐	☐
Quality and completeness of work performed	☐	☐	☐	☐	☐
Vehicle ready when promised	☐	☐	☐	☐	☐
Repair completed to your satisfaction the first time	☐	☐	☐	☐	☐

69

Also, notice the instructions. You learn that the real survey is going to be sent by someone else. You also learn that although you might have thought you were rating the entire organization, you are actually rating the person's personal performance, which becomes part of his personal record. If you don't feel he has earned an excellent rating, call and allow him to correct his shortcomings and failures. In other words, you could get him fired, it's implied, if you give him anything less than a perfect score.

Why does this automobile dealership do this? For the same reason hospitals are doing it. Bonuses are probably attached to getting the highest ratings in a region or state. Where there is competition for rewards or fear of consequences based on the numbers, people will naturally do whatever it takes to get high numbers as long as it cannot be construed as outright dishonest.

Rewards and punishments will help a company's scores go up, but at what price? Have their scores become more important than the truth? Will they go up because customer loyalty has gone up, or will they go up because competition and fear has motivated managers to figure out how to blur the line between satisfied and loyal to get customers to raise the score without raising their opinion?

HOSPITALS, TOO, ARE URGING HIGHER SCORES.

It is rapidly becoming common practice for hospitals trying to make a big push in service excellence to go over the survey at admission and urge the patient to either give fives or complain. Then after the patient is in a room, a nurse manager, often accompanied by another nurse, will visit each patient and emphasize the importance of giving fives on the nursing section of the survey or letting the nurse manager know what it would take to get fives. Finally, at discharge, the patient hears the same counsel one more time. I asked a director of nurses about this practice, and her response was, "It is just about the numbers. If we are held accountable for the numbers, and our bonuses are attached to the numbers, we will do what it takes to legally get those numbers. That's what the system rewards."

Unlike these hospitals I must say that no one at the car dealership put pressure on me face-to-face. When I arrived with my car and described my problem, the manager did not tell me all about the survey and how important it was for me to give him all fives. He didn't come into the waiting room and kneel down on one knee to go over the survey questionnaire with me once more. And he didn't go over my duty either to give fives or lodge an official complaint as I was paying my bill. At least the car dealership service department used the more gentle approach of a letter.

I first became aware of the practice of trying to induce a more favorable score from patients when a hospital attracted national attention by going from the lowest quartile in the Press Ganey *Patient-Satisfaction Survey* to the 98th percentile in little more than a year. Among the many commendable things they did to improve patient and employee loyalty, they instituted the practice of urging patients at several points in the process to give fives on survey questions unless they were willing to tell the staff how to improve enough to earn a five.

In 1999 the Healthcare Advisory Board presented its research on service excellence and best practices in service quality in hospitals. At their conferences where the research was presented, the question kept coming up from audiences about the practice of exhorting the patient either to give the highest score or to register a complaint. "Doesn't this skew the real meaning of the numbers?" people asked. The answer given was simply, "There is nothing inherently wrong about doing it." Nowhere was it suggested that this did not skew the scores. They readily agreed that this practice could push scores significantly higher than the patient would have given if not exhorted in this manner.

Make no mistake; this manipulation works. If we pressure people to inflate their ratings, they will do it. With this technique any hospital can effect a significant positive change in their scores overnight without doing anything differently to earn the scores. It may even place them in the highest percentile among hospitals collecting satisfaction scores. But, at what price is this reward achieved? Regrettably the price is self-induced blindness by creating a false sense of security in the one honest number that can protect its future–the percentage of loyal promoters.

PATIENT LOYALTY IS TOO IMPORTANT
TO BE BLURRED WITH SATISFACTION.

World-class service organizations like Disney count only the fives, but they do not try to make their fives say anything other than "very satisfied" on a scale that has two other numbers for those who are merely "satisfied." This is because they are genuinely trying to measure loyalty, not satisfaction. If knowing what percentage of your customers is highly likely to be loyal is important, why would an organization blur that distinction by trying to combine your loyal customers with your satisfied but not loyal customers?

Marriott uses a company that sends out surveys with a 10-point scale. Here the customers who give a 10 are considered highly likely to be loyal. Think of how much more difficult it is to get a 10 on a 10-point scale than a five on a five-point scale! And during your stay, there is no mention of a survey or coaching on how to respond. Marriott, like Disney, measures to improve, not to impress.

Frederick F. Reichheld, the world's leading authority on customer loyalty with his books, *Loyalty Rules* and *The Loyalty Effect*, has spent over a decade looking for the right questions with the right yardstick to determine customer and employee loyalty. In the December, 2003 issue of *Harvard Business Review*, he purports to have finally found it through exhaustive research involving 14 companies in 6 industries. The best question was, "How likely is it that you would recommend (company X) to a friend or colleague?" In order to reduce the effect of "grade inflation" inherent in 5 point scales, he and his researchers settled on a score where ten means "extremely likely" to recommend, five means neutral, and zero means "not at all likely." He goes on to explain:

> When we examined customer referral and repurchase behaviors along this scale we found three logical clusters. "Promoters," the customers with the highest rates of repurchase and referral, gave ratings of nine or ten to the question. The "passively satisfied" logged a seven or an eight, and "detractors" scored from zero to six...
>
> Not only did clustering customers into three categories...turn out to be the simplest, most intuitive, and best predictor of

customer behavior; it also made sense to frontline managers, who could relate to the goal of increasing the number of promoters and reducing the number of detractors more readily than increasing the mean of their satisfaction index by one standard deviation.[1]

A further refinement of this measurement system is to plot a company's "net promoters" as the one number a company needs to grow. He went on to describe what the research showed:

> Where we could obtain comparable and reliable revenue-growth data for a range of competitors, and where there were sufficient consumer responses, we plotted each firm's net promoters—the percentage of promoters minus the percentage of detractors—against the company's revenue growth rate.
>
> The results were striking. In airlines, for example, a strong correlation existed between net-promoter figures and a company's average growth rate over the three-year period from 1999 to 2002. Remarkably, this one simple statistic seemed to explain the relative growth rates across the entire industry; that is, no airline has found a way to increase growth without improving its ratio of promoters to detractors…"[2]

To my knowledge no hospital has risen to this level of scorekeeping yet. Most of them are still thinking as we thought back in 1985 at Florida Hospital: people are either satisfied or dissatisfied. We used to lump all the satisfied numbers (three, four, and five) together and essentially turn our five-point scale into a two-point scale. If you are going to do this, why have a five-point scale at all? Why not simply have Yes/No boxes beside questions like "Were you satisfied with your nursing care?"

It makes no sense to adopt scoring systems from the service leaders without adopting their rigor in protecting the subtle difference between customers who are highly likely to be loyal promoters of their services and those who are likely to defect, even though they said they were satisfied. They know their future depends on the honest difference in the customer's mind between satisfaction and loyalty.

PATIENTS HAVE NO COMPLAINTS
WHEN THEY ARE SATISFIED.

I can hear some hospital administrators saying, "We do not do this to inflate our numbers. We do it to get patients to speak up about their care. How will we learn how to improve if we do not ask them to tell us?"

Regarding the first statement, I would say that anything that pressures the score-giver into giving a higher response is done for the sole purpose of inflating the numbers. This practice is manipulative because a satisfied person *has no complaints*! To insist that he or she complain or give a perfect score forces the shades of meaning intended by a five-point scale into a simple Yes/No response. They may have had an ordinary experience in which nobody went out of his or her way to establish a warm relationship, but nobody did anything *wrong* either. Then someone comes along and suggests in the name of feedback that since the patient cannot think of anything anyone did wrong, the patient is obliged to give the highest score. That will probably get the desired five, but it distorts the meaning of the numbers and effectively negates the patient's true feelings.

To the second and third statements above, I would say that you can get feedback about how to improve your services simply by asking a question like, "Was there anything frustrating or disappointing about your experience?" During admission tell patients and their families how to complain if anything does not meet with their satisfaction. Nursing managers can still make rounds and ask, "How are we treating you? What would make your stay better?" And during the discharge process there is nothing wrong with asking if their stay was satisfactory or could have been better, just as most fine restaurants do as you pay your bill.

The issue is not with asking for feedback from patients and visitors; it is with our trying to influence their responses to make us look better. When our goal is to look better, we are measuring to impress, not to improve. If our motive is to get honest feedback, why not be like Disney and Marriott and avoid bringing up the survey at all?

Much of what it takes to create loyalty is beyond what can be specifically required of employees. Competence and courtesy are expected and should be equally hardwired into staff behavior. But meeting these expectations does not automatically produce a loyal patient because they expect any hospital to do the same. It isn't meeting patients' expectations that makes a stay unique or special. It is the spontaneous, unexpected, memorable moments that generate feelings of loyalty. More often than not, it is the compassionate connection between a caregiver and a patient that elevates common courtesy into something more tender and unforgettable than good, routine care. Insisting that a person be able to tell you what it takes to change an ordinary experience into an extraordinary one is asking for more than the responder can give. People do not know what it takes to turn what they expect into something *more* than they expect. The reason such events become stories is precisely that the patient was *surprised* by what happened. How can one tell someone else what would surprise them?

In the light of this concept, let's revisit some of the previous stories I have told:

There was the Chinese restaurant that satisfied me in every respect but didn't have my undivided loyalty until they discovered how to obtain a product I didn't even know existed in America. How could I have told them what it would take to earn my loyalty? They had to discover that on their own and surprise me.

Then there was Judy, whose nurse held her hand late one lonely night as she wept. It changed Judy from a satisfied patient into a loyal patient, but how could she have lodged a complaint if this had not happened? Could Judy have said, "If you want a five on your survey from me, I need nurses to hold my hand when I cry"? Of course not. It takes something personal and heartfelt, not something routine, to make a loyal patient. Patients can't possibly know how to ask for such things, but they surely know how to respond when they happen—with fives and their enthusiastic loyalty.

My stay at the Residence Inn by Marriott was perfect as far as I could tell, but I was not particularly loyal until someone from the maintenance department cleaned my windshield on a cold November morning. If they had asked me how to improve their hotel services I would not have been able to think of anything. What earned my loyalty was something I would never have been able to tell them, much less complain about not getting! They had to come up with it themselves and pleasantly surprise me.

One of the things that impressed me during a hospital stay was having a white dry-erase board on the wall at the foot of my bed. At the beginning of each shift, my nurse would come in and write her name and the name of her assistant on the board in big letters so I could easily read them. I had never seen this done before, but I loved it. It made me think these nurses were special because they did something I did not expect. It changed an ordinary satisfied rating into a five. If they did not have these boards and put pressure on me to tell them what it would take to get my highest rating, how could I have come up with something I had never heard of before? All I would be able to do is give them a score they were pressuring me to give.

Remember, customers can tell you only what they have come to expect. But what they expect is also what they consider ordinary. They cannot tell you what extraordinary looks like. That takes commitment, empathy, and creativity on the part of administrators, managers, and caregivers. Surprise them with kindness. Surprise them with empathy. Surprise them with innovations. Surprise them with something extraordinary, and you will earn their undivided loyalty.

Patient loyalty is far more important than a numbers game, because the difference between satisfaction and loyalty is the difference between fool's gold and something you can take to the bank to protect your future against competitive forces. Turning the gold of patient loyalty into the fool's gold of satisfaction is a confusing, if not dangerous, game.

IF YOU WANT THE TRUTH, ASK THE HOUSEKEEPERS.

Anyone who saw the movie *A Few Good Men* will never forget the powerful courtroom scene at the climax of the film when Tom Cruise is pressing Jack Nicholson, a military officer, to tell the truth. "You want the truth?" Nicholson snaps. "You can't *handle* the truth."

I sometimes think of these words when healthcare administrators talk about getting and measuring patient feedback—especially if I know that the feedback is collected only once or twice a year; or when the feedback is used only to compare themselves with other hospitals in the system; or when patient-satisfaction scores are largely unknown by the staff; or when the return on the random sample is too small to be significant; or when no money is spent on personal callbacks or focus groups with recently discharged patients to learn about their experience; or when the survey results do not generate any action other than trying to game the numbers by making it look like they are saying something better than they are.

What would a serious attempt to get patient feedback look like? It would need to have four primary requisites:

1. It would seek to get the most honest response possible.
2. It would be gathered immediately, while the patient was still in the hospital, and again right after discharge while the experience is still fresh in the mind and the staff can take action as soon as possible.
3. It would be statistically valid and reliable.
4. It would encourage comments and specific examples.

For many years we have known from numerous experiments conducted by social psychologists that there is a negative correlation between the perceived status of a questioner and the willingness of the respondent to be open and honest. In other words, when it comes to sensitive content, a psychiatric resident is more likely to get the patient to talk about things that are embarrassing to talk about than the chief psychiatrist. A person in a position of authority is less likely to get honest, but negative, comments than a person with no authority. A person in a lab coat will more likely get what the respondent thinks he is looking for than the truth. A nurse may learn things the physician didn't pick up because the patient didn't want to look dumb in front of the physician.

Most of us can relate to this research intuitively. Let's imagine a typical, elderly woman who is a patient in the hospital. Let's assume that she has a complaint that she is afraid to express. Maybe she feels that one of her night nurses is rude and has made some condescending comments to her about her lifestyle relating to her condition. How are we going to get this patient to speak up about this sensitive issue and give us a chance to deal with the insensitive nurse? Certainly not by waiting for six months and hoping our random sample of surveyed patients will catch it. We know we need to get this kind of information while the patient is in the hospital. As my friend Dave Buker, a total quality management consultant and trainer, says, "It's not how soon you hear the good news that matters; it's how soon you hear the bad news." Some method of real-time feedback needs to be implemented.

Let's imagine that we have decided that a member of the hospital staff will be trained to elicit vital information from patients. Who among the following is more likely to get the unvarnished truth: the hospital administrator, the director of nurses, the head nurse, or a housekeeper? Intuition would tell us that it would be the housekeeper, especially if he or she has been taught to be friendly and ask how things are going. Why? Because the housekeeper has the lowest perceived status. The person least likely to get an honest response to the question "How is everybody treating you?" is probably the administrator.

When I was a vice president at Florida Hospital, for a short time we instituted something we called SHARE visits. Each vice president was expected to visit several patients a week in their rooms and ask how things were going. About all we learned from these visits was that people were exceptionally happy with their care. There were virtually no complaints. The program withered because it quickly became viewed as a waste of time for busy vice presidents.

After doing this for a while, I began to wonder if patients were telling me the truth. I remember going into a room and introducing myself to a man who was the patient and his wife who was visiting. He seemed to be too incapacitated to carry on a conversation, so I asked her how things were going. She raved about how wonderful the nurses were, how great the hospital was, how they loved us. Then I decided to probe harder than usual. I said, "It's wonderful to hear that you appreciate our staff, but it's hard for me to believe that we are perfect. Surely you have encountered *some* frustrations. That's what I really want to hear about. I am more interested in how we can improve than in how good we are."

She started to reassure me again, but it sounded a little weaker than the first comments, so I just stood there. There was a stirring in the bed and her husband mumbled something. "I guess we did have a discouraging morning," she said. "They got my husband up and around before breakfast for a seven o'clock appointment in the cath lab. When we got down there, we were told that he was not on their schedule. They seemed upset that we had shown up unexpectedly and treated us as if it were our fault. They kept us there for the entire morning, telling us that they were going to work us in. Finally they gave up and sent him back to his room, but by now lunch was gone and they couldn't get him a lunch tray. So here he is hungry, without a bite to eat all day, and still no procedure done."

This sounded like a serious complaint to me! But what became painfully clear was how reluctant many people are to complain to a person in a position of authority. After that I saw that having senior leadership visit patients in their rooms might be good public relations, but it is not the most effective way to unearth dissatisfaction or patient-experience problems.

I have often wondered about developing a systematic way of having people who are perceived to have low status or no authority seek out complaints. Knowing the reluctance of patients to express dissatisfaction, I don't think it is too farfetched an idea to train housekeepers—or volunteers—to help be the eyes and ears for spontaneous patient feedback. They would have to collaborate with nursing and be trained in the proper asking etiquette. They would need to learn how to empathize with the patient and ask for permission to pass on the information to the right people. Then they would need to know who gets the information and in what way. Finally, there would need to be a system for collecting, tracking, and acting on the information that is gathered. Unless these steps are all in place—the steps for actual improvement—the information should not be collected in person at the bedside by anybody.

DISCHARGE PHONE CALLS HAVE A POWERFUL EFFECT.

In my experience there is nothing quite as powerful in influencing patient-satisfaction scores legitimately as discharge phone calls. This is where a nurse who cared for the patient calls the patient within a day or two of discharge to ask how things are going. Every now and then a nursing director will express dismay over getting higher scores from surgery patients than general medical patients, yet they are cared for by the same nurses and are often more difficult patients. My first response is "Do you make callbacks to your surgery patients?" The answer is almost always "Yes." Then I ask if they do the same for their non-surgical patients. The answer is almost always "No."

The patients are not finished with a hospital until they are well, or as well as they are going to be. Since hospitals send people home before they are well due to reimbursement policies, technically the patient is not finished yet. Discharge instructions are often long and complicated. They tell patients how to take care of themselves at home for the duration of the healing process. Often these instructions seem clear to the patient when listening to the discharge nurse but become quite confusing when they try to implement them at home. Imagine how reassuring it is to get a call from the nurse a day later, asking if everything is going well and getting a chance to ask questions and clarify concerns.

The perfect time to solicit feedback on a patient's overall experience is when the patient is doing well on discharge and has no further questions about their medical care. Just the asking will be seen as caring, even compassionate. The feedback on satisfaction will be immediate. If the patient points out something that didn't go right, it can be addressed right away and reported back to the patient.

A discharge phone call is not a marketing task added to a nurse's load. It is an integral part of the patient's care. Caregivers need to see that continuation of care extends to the home more than ever in today's healthcare environment. The patient does not really have closure with the hospital or their clinical care until recovery at home has been completed. No wonder hospitals that do discharge phone calls on every patient generally get higher scores on patient satisfaction and loyalty than hospitals that don't.

INTERNAL DEPARTMENTS NEED TO GET FEEDBACK TOO.

A score or more companies offer patient satisfaction surveys for hospitals. By the time this book is published, there will likely be a national survey conducted by the government on all Medicare and

Medicaid patients. While frontline caregivers are being rated by patients, numerous departments are not measured because they do not interface directly with patients. They may not be serving the patient, but they are serving coworkers who do. If measuring performance as viewed through the customer's eyes is important for patients who are customers, why not nurses who are internal customers? If "what gets noticed gets done," as the adage goes, and dimensions of service are important, internal support services need to receive feedback from their customers as well. If presented in the right way, it can provide measurement that helps motivate employees and improve performance.

The overarching purpose for collecting feedback is for a team and its individual members to gauge and track their own performance, not to provide a stick for top management. This means that the team should play the main role in leading out and designing the measurement process and tools. The tool should be simple and accurate and not try to measure more than a handful of things: the major things that matter to their customers. I usually insist that at least one question has to do with courtesy, since customers will not likely mention courtesy as a key indicator of quality, but they are certainly offended when it is absent.

It is important that teams have the conversations they need to develop their own system of getting feedback and showing their measurement in graphical form. To help facilitate that conversation, here are some good questions to help them get started:

1. Who are our customers for each service we offer?
2. Is it important *to our team* to meet their needs and wants?
3. Do we know what their needs and wants are? How can we be sure?
4. How can we know we are meeting their needs and wants?
5. How can we get an accurate picture of our performance in their eyes?
6. How will we use the information for improvement?
7. How will we know we are improving?
8. Will it be timely?
9. Will it be easy to understand and use?

Nurses have found that making rounds on patient floors to talk to patients while they are in the hospital and calling them after discharge is a highly effective way to learn about patient needs and satisfaction. It also provides an opportunity to solve problems and pass on compliments. The power and effectiveness of this personal information gathering cannot be overstated and provides a good example of what other departments could be doing on a regular basis also.

The benefits associated with improving service, generating goodwill, problem solving, and passing on compliments can all be realized simply by scheduling regular visits by department managers to nursing units. Food service can learn about how the food is being delivered and problems that might be part of the process. Pharmacists would be able to eliminate one of the most common sources of friction in hospitals by visiting nursing units and talking with nurses about their frustrations with medications. The same could be said for housekeeping, engineering, information services, and almost every other department. And it creates a culture of soliciting feedback to improve, not to impress. Besides, no amount of quantifiable numbers will ever have as much impact on behavior as anecdotal information about a department's performance.

---

1. Frederick R. Reichheld, *The One Number You Need to Grow,* Harvard Business Review, December 2003, p. 51.
2. Ibid.

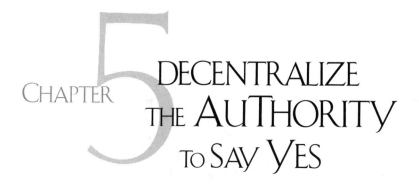

CHAPTER 5

DECENTRALIZE THE AUTHORITY TO SAY YES

Not long ago, I was invited to conduct a series of customer relations training sessions for frontline employees at one of the satellite hospitals of a large hospital system. Several days had gone along without a hitch. But then, on one particular morning, the classroom door was locked when I arrived. I looked in the windows and could see that the classroom had not been set up for instruction. Chairs were scattered all over the room and the tables were stacked and pushed against the walls.

A small group of early attendees began to gather outside the door. I asked how to get in but nobody knew. One person volunteered to go to administration and ask. She returned to say that the administrative offices were still closed. We called environmental services, but they did not have a key to the classroom. We called security. A security officer arrived with a passkey but insisted that he did not have the authority to open the room.

"But you can see we are all here for the class," I said. "Weren't you in this class yesterday?"

"Yes, I know," he answered. "But I am not allowed to open a room without permission to do so from central dispatch."

"Maybe there is somebody in administration by now," I ventured.

"That won't do any good," he said. "I don't take orders from administration. I have to call my dispatch office, which is across town at the main hospital. Until they tell me to open the classroom, I can't. I'm really sorry."

In due time the classroom was opened, but from my point of view, the point of view of a guest, security had a system that made no sense. How could central dispatch, 20 miles away, have a better understanding of the situation than the officer at the scene? Any information about the problem would be coming from the officer anyway. What possible knowledge could central dispatch bring to bear that would make their judgment in this case more sound than that of their frontline person?

At another one of the hospitals in this same system, I happened to tell this experience to an executive I knew quite well. She laughed. "I had a doctor once who had left something in the medical library," she told me, "but even I couldn't get the guy from security, a guy I knew really well, to open the door so this doctor could get his stuff. He said he had to wait for orders from their central office across town."

Here is an example of a functional silo, spread across a metropolitan area, that gives its employees only the ability to say, "No," or at best, "Please wait for me to get permission," even to administrators. If anybody, internal or external, needs service, he must go through central control. The people at the top of the silo are the only ones with the authority to say "Yes."

DISNEY DISMANTLED FUNCTIONAL SILOS.

Through the years Disney has been able to be more responsive to guests and create more empowered cast members by dismantling functional silos and pushing decision making and problem solving closer to the front lines. Many organizations talk about doing the same thing, but few are able to carry it out.

Take EPCOT Center for example. It is a theme park laid out in a figure 8 with the top circle of the 8 forming a lake. Around the perimeter of the lake are pavilions representing different countries of the world. In each of these pavilions there is a show for education and entertainment, a restaurant or concession serving food, and a shop for

selling merchandise. Each of these three functions was like
service, a silo with its own cost-revenue center and its ow
All the restaurants in all the pavilions were under one
authority. All the merchandising in all the facilities were und... another
authority. The general manager of the pavilion did not have any
authority over employees from the other functions. If a special show on
tour from overseas needed some extra space, the pavilion manager was
unable to move some merchandise or a concession stand without
permission. If merchandising had a big new item to push, they couldn't
get floor space on the general manager's turf or in the restaurant for
advertising, because that was somebody else's territory.

In a major reorganization of its structure in the eighties, Disney
eliminated a significant amount of bureaucracy by putting everything
that goes on at each pavilion under one cost center. All the employees
reported to one general manager who could make things happen in the
interest of what was best for customer service and the bottom line *at
that location*, which now included *all* functions. There was still a central
place that provided merchandise and another that ordered and shipped
food supplies to them, but the actual service and the cast members that
provided that service were all accountable to one general manager.

One of the managers told me how this affected the staff. "We really
work like a team now because we have one focus and that is the success
of our pavilion. We all get behind whatever makes sense in terms of
more revenue or better service at our show, and everyone
enthusiastically makes it happen. One of the best things about being on
one team, instead of three or four, is our ability to cross-train and cross-
utilize all the cast members who work here. This allows people to do
many different jobs in our area instead of only one. It relieves boredom,
keeps them fresh, and helps them see how their jobs affect others.
Another payoff that we didn't expect is getting a lot more ideas and
suggestions than we ever got before. The change this reorganization has
made in our area is really dramatic, and everybody loves it."

On a wall backstage at one of Disney's resorts, I saw a large sign
with a list of value statements for cast members that could be read all
the way down the hall. The statement that surprised me said: "You are
always right when satisfying a guest." If you come late or miss a meeting

...ause you're trying to serve a guest, you're exonerated. If you decide to buy something from the gift shop to placate an upset guest, you are not going to be reprimanded for spending too much. A value statement like this clearly empowers people to say Yes to a guest's request instead of passing the decision up the line to a supervisor. And it's on the wall backstage for all employees to read day in and day out.

DISNEY DECENTRALIZED SERVICE RECOVERY.

When EPCOT Center opened, there was a guest services office not far from the main entrance. If something happened to a guest that shouldn't have happened, the unhappy person was sent to the guest services center. If it happened at the American Pavilion, the show that was the farthest away, it was a very long walk just to be heard and have a problem addressed. The only people who could give recovery (a gift with an apology to regain the guest's goodwill) were the people in this central office.

During the time when the silos were reorganized, Disney decentralized the guest services function as well. If a guest had a problem at the American Pavilion, he or she would be able to see a service manager on duty at that pavilion who could offer service recovery.

This was a big improvement, but compared to a company like Nordstrom, it was not the benchmark in responsiveness and service recovery. Nordstrom stories created a legendary image of a retailer whose employees were empowered to offer service recovery on the spot. They could give away merchandise or take cash out of registers without checking with anyone. Customers loved it so much that their word of mouth created an avalanche of publicity and loyalty for Nordstrom worth untold millions of dollars.

Not to be outdone, Disney followed suit. The power to say Yes in service recovery was passed on to frontline cast members. After some training in the process and the wide variety of situations and recovery options available to them, cast members could offer whatever seemed fair, from an ice cream cone to several nights stay in an expensive resort. They were given the power to give away a valuable gift on the spot if needed. That's spontaneity with real authority based on trust ιι member's judgment!

Terry Barter, director of rehabilitation services at Florida Hospital, says that autonomy and decision making are keys to retaining excellent staff. "Being micromanaged by one's boss is the surest way to lose talented people," he says. He told about a therapist who had a very upset patient who weighed over 400 pounds. Evidently the only oversized walker the department owned for extremely obese patients was being used by another patient. Instead of telling the patient to wait for the walker to be turned in, the therapist, in the name of good customer service and recovery, went out immediately and bought a larger walker with his own money. Barter said he was pleased that the therapist took responsibility. Instead of calling his supervisor, he acted on his own, knowing his decision would be supported. And because he acted so quickly, the patient was pleased as well.

The authority to say Yes elevates the status of every employee. A major contributor to burnout is a feeling that one has no control over one's work. Being unable to make decisions, unable to please a patient or the family without permission, unable to do anything but pass on complaints, is debilitating and discouraging. It becomes even worse when managers insist that their employees say No only to overrule the employee when the complaint comes to them. Think how demoralizing it must be for the security officer to be unable to perform a simple task spontaneously, especially if 10 minutes later he is instructed to do the thing he would have done anyway. Only now he looks stupid and ineffective to the customer. Multiply this embarrassment and lack of autonomy by many events in a day, and we are faced with the turnover of excellent employees.

Once, years ago, when I was the administrator on call, I got paged while I was in church. I went out to a phone and called the switchboard operator who said she had a very upset physician who wanted to talk to me. The physician came on the line and related how he had been called in on his day off by the emergency department to assess a critical case. As he was leaving, his car ran out of gas right in the emergency parking lot. He said, "Nobody seems to be able to give me a hand here. I tried security, but the guy says he is the only one here and can't reach

nission to leave the premises and take me to a nearby
perator then paged the engineer on call, and he took
down, only to say it wasn't his job. He said he thought
y's job. Can't anybody around here perform a simple act

I said, "...m awfully sorry. Where is the security person?"

"Right here."

"Let me speak to him." He put the person on, and when I got his name, I simply said, "Dan, this physician has been frustrated for nearly an hour trying to get some help with his car. I'm sure you'd like to help him, but I understand you feel you need permission to leave the campus for a few minutes, so I'm giving you permission. Would you please get a container from engineering and go get him some gasoline. Get a receipt. Don't let the physician pay for it. Apologize profusely and then send me the receipt. I'll make sure you get reimbursed."

Think of how this young man would have felt if he had been able to do all this on his own without permission. He would have felt like a manager. Empowered. Helpful. Effective. Probably even inspired. And think how pleased the physician would have made him feel in the process. What a different ending it would have been. By the time a manager or a vice president has to step in to make something commonsense happen for the customer, nobody wins. The customer is not impressed. In that very act, we lost our chance to shine. Only frontline people can shine in such situations; managers cannot. Unless we shine in problem situations, we cannot gain the customer's loyalty.

The centralized authority to say Yes may come from the need to be organized and consistent, but, paradoxically the result is that to the customer it appears to be just the opposite. Besides, it creates a culture of dependency, which is at the root of bureaucratic organizations. Surely this is the kind of organization Ralph Waldo Emerson meant when he wrote, "A foolish consistency is the hobgoblin of little minds, adored by little statesmen" (or, we might say, *little managers*). We rarely hear quoted the end of Emerson's thought: "With consistency a great soul has simply nothing to do." That is the heart of the matter. When one person makes all the decisions in the name of consistency, great souls, our best employees, are demeaned to the level of robots and we rob them of the joy of autonomy and the growth that comes from the practice of sound judgment.

Structure drives culture.

Many hospitals are hampered by the same centralized structure that used to plague Disney, and may even still plague Disney in some of its operations. The incessant creep of centralization under insecure managers without the confidence to delegate and dependent workers who are powerless is pervasive. In some healthcare systems satellite hospital administrators have little control over their own emergency departments or the staff that runs them. They don't really own their own security, or purchasing, or X-ray, or human resources, or any number of other so-called departments. These departments are all extensions of a larger corporate structure. Everything has to come from headquarters, where every request is scrutinized, restudied, and second-guessed by people who are almost never on site. Service can get so poor and communications so slow that the whole culture becomes inoculated against speed and responsiveness. The only way to get anything done quickly is to work around the system. And our key attribute, *spontaneity*, if it ever existed before centralization, quickly evaporates.

Structure drives culture. It is not possible to create a world-class service culture as long as we keep structures that are defined by layers of bureaucracy and departmental barriers to speed and responsiveness. The most important single change that can accompany a strong service message is spontaneity, the power of inspired frontline staff to say Yes and do the fair or generous thing on the spot.

The title of chapter 2, "Make Courtesy More Important Than Efficiency," is a key principle that might appear on a poster somewhere, but most hospital departments do not support this principle with their structure. Managers teach and reward just the opposite in their training and evaluations. Employees who act on the principle of courtesy over efficiency are likely to find themselves on the red carpet.

A secretary who starts to take work orders over the phone when the structure is that they must always be sent in on the proper form through proper channels will soon be reprimanded.

A clerk in accounting who does someone a favor by making out a check for reimbursement before the required cycle time had better not do it too often.

A nurse who makes an exception to some rule for a family visiting from another state might have to apologize to her manager.

A cashier who opens the cash register in the cafeteria between meals to help an exhausted family that has been in the emergency room all day with no food believes she might get into trouble because technically the cafeteria is closed.

A security guard who unlocks the door to the medical library for a physician may have to say, "I'm not supposed to do this, so don't tell anyone."

And everywhere we keep hearing phrases like "I don't know." Or "That's not my job." Or "My supervisor is gone right now; you'll have to talk to her." Or "We can't do that." Or "I didn't make the rules!" Or "It isn't my fault."

It is senseless to teach frontline people in a service-excellence class not to say these things if our structure ties their hands so they are forced to say them. Changing *how* we say No might get us an inch toward better service, but changing the management systems so we *can* say Yes will get us a mile by comparison. I suppose it is easier to teach employees to *sound* more responsible, than actually empowering them to *be* responsible. But without real authority the customer usually sees through the talk and judges the organization by the walk.

CYNICISM RESULTS FROM WEAK IMPLEMENTATION.

If an organization tries to instill a service culture through a program, it will raise everyone's expectation that they will be empowered to give better service by managers, who will demonstrate how it is done in their departments. This is trouble in the making if the structures remain that make it difficult to give great service in the first place. Many hospitals have tried this approach with sincere determination, some two or three times, and all it has done in the end is to create indifference—and even hostility—to such programs. The cynicism left in the wake of superficial efforts to change culture through banners, exhortations, and training programs is palpable. I have seen it and felt it many times during the assessment phase of trying to determine if an organization is ready for what it will take to make deep change.

What typically happens is what social psychologists call the "inoculation theory." Inoculation is giving a small dose of a weak virus that is fought off by the body's natural resistance, so that any chance of a "take" when exposed to a strong version of the real thing is effectively prevented. This happens in the psychological world of attitudes and beliefs as well. When the structure of the organization quietly repels the "virus" of service-excellence training, and all the optimism generated in the beginning dissipates, it is almost impossible for that organization ever to be "infected" with a full-blown commitment to those ideas and attitudes in the future. The antibody of cynicism is too pervasive. Middle managers become inoculated. They like to say they could have told you it wouldn't work in the first place. The efficiency experts will point out how much time and money was wasted. Finance will show that nothing improved on the bottom line. Marketing will find no evidence that there has been significant improvement in patient satisfaction or gain in market share. What are the chances of becoming a great service organization after a management structure has successfully warded off its most salient characteristics: speed, responsiveness, and spontaneity?

The worst part about it is that the *program* will be blamed, not the management systems and structures in the organization that effectively killed it. The people who run the departments will look out their windows at the teachers and trainers and shake their heads, instead of looking in the mirror and saying, "How did I and my policies contribute to the demise of an important opportunity for our organization to become great?"

For some reason the talented people who are given the responsibility for creating and implementing the desired culture are not the same people who have the authority to change the organization's policies and procedures, or the complicated management systems that typify most large departments.

WHO IS TO BLAME WHEN A
SERVICE EXCELLENCE PROGRAM FAILS?

When I started out to learn as much as I could about transformational leadership, total quality management, organizational culture, and customer loyalty, I held a bias that was shared in much of the literature of the eighties and nineties. Namely, if it doesn't work, it must be the fault of top management. Unless the people at the top, especially the CEO and VPs, lead the way and make it happen with relentless focus, it will die. Employees are not empowered because managers will not let go of control, and when efforts to meet customer needs and wants go nowhere, it's easy to think it's because these efforts are not being supported by top management.

I am not as certain about these views any longer. I now believe the blame for slowness and lack of responsiveness is rarely the fault of the president or CEO. It is not the decisions at the very top that hamper the delivery of good service. It is often all the decisions in the layers below it, starting with vice presidents.

In thinking back over the stories and illustrations I have used in this book, both good and bad, I cannot think of one that has anything to do with top management. Let's take the example that led off this chapter about the inability of the security guard to say Yes. How did his lack of authority have anything to do with top management?

You might say, "Well, top management probably creates a command and control culture that all the other managers are expected to imitate." But in this case, and probably most others, I don't think that fits the facts. A good illustration occurred the very next day, after the locked classroom incident, at the same facility, in the same hospital system.

I decided to get to this hospital early to make sure the classroom was unlocked, which it was. Since everything was set up the way I wanted it, I had enough time to eat breakfast in the cafeteria. When I tasted the breakfast potatoes, I moaned audibly at how delicious they were. I couldn't remember when I had eaten such savory potatoes. How in the world did they get them so crunchy and moist at the same time? And what was that extra flavor that excited my taste buds? I decided I had to ask somebody how they were made. I pictured myself making them at home for some guests.

When I went back toward the kitchen, I saw the food service director of all the hospitals in the entire system. She was dressed in the business attire of an executive. She is the one who tells all the other hospital cafeterias how to do their jobs, what they can serve, and what they can't serve. She hires and fires managers, writes policy, and dictates menu selections. She has been a director for years, training cooks, teaching quality control, and expanding food service–the perfect person to ask.

I was surprised when she told me she did not know how the potatoes were made. If they were so good, she certainly wanted to know how the cook had done it. She went to the kitchen while I waited. When she returned she had the cook in tow, a young woman in a white uniform and a hair net, flushed with nervousness. She seemed relieved when I said, "Your potatoes are just wonderful. Do you bake them first or do you boil them first? Or do you just fry them or broil them raw? And what do you put on them for that flavor? I want to be able to make these at home."

After the cook answered all my questions, I thanked her. She left, beaming with satisfaction, and I was smiling too. What I took away from that encounter was more than a recipe for potatoes. I saw how empowered a frontline cook was. I saw the pride she experienced in being able to share her recipe, not only with a customer, but with the head honcho herself! This was not a department hampered with micromanagement and excessive control. It was a department that provided guidelines but allowed spontaneity, creativity, and customer service to flourish.

The point of relating this experience is that the silo of food service is in the same corporate organization as the security silo. But the management culture and structure *within* the silos seemed much different.

Before I lay all the blame at the feet of managers, I should also say that many employees do not want the responsibility of deciding when to say Yes and when to say No. They do not want to be empowered. They say things to their managers like "Don't ask me to do that. That's what they pay you the big bucks for." Over time, however, I would expect an empowering manager to have weeded these people out and created a team of people eager to take responsibility.

Jack Welch, the highly admired former CEO of General Electric, has distilled his management philosophy into three values: speed, simplicity, and self-confidence. Speed is the essential measure of productivity. Simplicity is the essential characteristic of good communication and structure. And self-confidence is the primary quality of a good leader. He goes on to point out that it takes comprehensive knowledge plus self-confidence for a manager to simplify the complexities of ideas, decisions, and systems. It also takes self-confidence to push decision making to the front so that speed, the test of productivity, can take place. To paraphrase something my friend Dave Buker, a performance-improvement consultant to Fortune 500 companies, says, "First-rate managers hire first-rate people and turn them loose. Second-rate managers hire third-rate people who have to be told what to do and how to do it."

I believe Jack Welch is right. The reason some managers cannot let go is that they are insecure. A vice president once said to me: "I admit that I am a control freak, but I work rings around everyone else in administration. I am the first one here in the morning and I am the last to leave. I am in constant touch with all my departments. I am on top of the details. So what if I'm a workaholic. I take that as a compliment. If my people don't like it, they can go work for somebody else."

While he was talking, I thought to myself, *Yes, but it's because you lack self-confidence that you do these things. Over time all the capable, talented, self-confident people will resent being micromanaged and leave.* This VP will keep the ones who are equally insecure, but who demonstrate it by being dependent instead of controlling. They just want to punch the time clock and do exactly what they're told. No decision making for them. It is the perfect codependent marriage of control and submissiveness, both rooted in lack of self-confidence. Great leaders are confident enough to hire talented, self-confident people and turn them loose.

Years ago I came across an unforgettable illustration that I have shared many times. Steve Brown, who was president of the Fortune Group, tells it in his excellent book, *13 Fatal Errors Managers Make and How You Can Avoid Them*. He had been asked to analyze and help solve a problem by the president of a real estate company with 27 branches in the Chicago area. Together they had more than 500 salespeople.

The president said, "I would like to have you talk with one of our managers. It seems our business is not his vocation. Our business is his avocation; his vocation is cards."

I pressed for details and he said, "He shows up at his office and spends about an hour-and-a-half in the morning before going across the street to the country club where he plays cards all day long. Then he returns to the office and spends about an hour before going home."

"Dick, before I talk with him, tell me about his office. For starters, among your 27 branches, where is his?"

"Oh, it's the largest."

"What about volume of business?"

"His office does more than any other branch."

"What about bottom-line profit?"

"Oh, it's our most profitable."

I thought we might have a case of a person spending a lifetime building a branch and deciding to semi-retire himself at full salary, so I added, "Well, what about growth?"

Dick said, "Percentage wise, it grows more than any of the others. There's hardly any turnover among his salespeople, and they absolutely love him."

Then Dick sighed, "Steve, what do you think we ought to do?"

I said, "I think we ought to find 27 more just like him. He's the best executive in the bunch!"[1]

The author goes on to say that a manager's success is not measured by what he can do, but by what his people can do without him.

Following years of effort trying to create learning organizations, Peter Senge has come to the same conclusion about assigning blame to top management for failed programs. For those of us who tend to blame top management for its lack of commitment or support, he offers some contrary assertions that also have the ring of truth.

We should be suspicious of the tendency of people in organizations to "look upward" and expect top management to fix things.

Little significant change can occur if it is driven from the top.

CEO proclamations and programs rolled out from corporate headquarters are a good way to undermine deeper changes.

Top-management 'buy-in' is a poor substitute for genuine commitment at many levels in an organization, and in fact, if management authority is used unwisely, it can make such commitment less rather than more likely.

Organizational surveys and focus groups, by focusing attention on "telling" top management what is wrong, can block learning because they do nothing to encourage individual accountability and tend to reinforce the mindset that only top management has the power to fix problems.[2]

I often do focus groups to gain a quick understanding of the culture from the point of view of middle managers. Sometimes I ask the question: "What do you see as barriers to service excellence?"

In one of these groups a manager responded by saying "Top management."

Another manager challenged the remark by asking, "How is top management a barrier to service excellence? Do I need top management's support to treat people nice? Do I need their support before I will greet everybody with a smile every day? Do I need their support before I can show compassion to someone or reassure a person who is waiting in the waiting area?"

I would add, Do we need top management's support to give more authority to frontline people to say Yes?

Granted, it is a big help when top management role models these behaviors, and it certainly appears incongruous when they don't. But a confident manager with a vision for service is rarely thwarted from doing them by top management.

Top management can articulate the vision and ask for measurable results. Energy, knowledge, problem solving, and implementation must come from inside the management ranks.

SERVICE RECOVERY IS THE TRUE TEST OF DECENTRALIZING.

The truest test of accountability is the degree to which someone can say Yes when it involves money. Giving frontline employees the power to make restitution, or buy a gift, or promise to write-off an item on a person's bill, is heady responsibility.

I have seen hospitals try to implement a service-recovery program from the top. Not many such programs seem to work for very long. When top management bypasses the department heads by trying to give the power of service recovery directly to frontline employees, resistance appears to sabotage it for several reasons:

1. Most service problems happen in the context of someone's department. An hourly employee isn't usually able to go around department procedures unless his or her boss says so. Even top management is unable to circumvent what is seen as the legitimate control of a middle manager.

2. Mistakes made in clinical departments have clinical ramifications that are far more complex than problems in a retail store, where returning the merchandise or being given a generous exchange will regain loyalty.

3. When bills are paid or partially paid by an insurance company, write-offs and restitution actually reward the insurance company, not the patient.

4. Department managers resent anything that takes them out of the loop in deciding what to do about a dissatisfied patient. Having top management fund recovery out of a special budget in administration without their input makes department heads feel undercut. Instead of seeing it as empowering, they see it as robbing them of their own empowerment. Besides, it should come out of their budget so that they will pay better attention to the cost of recovery and make it more obvious that preventive measures need to be put in place.

5. Departmental walls in hospitals are as sturdy as ever. Most of us have not gotten to the place where an employee from one department can initiate actions affecting the costs of another department.

6. Only by department can we install recovery systems that get triggered automatically, so that we do not reward only those who complain.

Service recovery, then, gives us another example of how the full support and even enthusiasm of top management cannot bring about employee empowerment. So does this mean service recovery is something that makes no sense in hospitals? Is it a concept that doesn't fit our work environment? No. I think it means that unilateral service recovery from administration doesn't work very well. Under a hospital-wide initiative, each department should be required to implement its own service standards. Recovery policies are simply part of those standards and procedures.

Often I tell a story about Nordstrom, which was told to me by someone who heard me speak. The lady got her shoe caught in an escalator in a Nordstrom store in California. As she stumbled off the escalator, a clerk rushed over to help her. When she had gotten the customer seated, she went back and retrieved the lady's high heel that had broken off. She also opened a package of new slippers and handed them to the lady with an apology for what happened. In most stores in those days, that would have been considered generous. But then the clerk asked for the lady's shoes and said, "Shop around here for a few minutes and let me see if the shoe department can do anything about this heel."

When the clerk returned from the shoe department, she had a new pair of expensive shoes, matched to the color and size of the customer's old ones. With a smile (and if you could give this kind of service, who wouldn't smile!) she told the customer that the new shoes were on the house. "If these aren't quite right, I'll take you to the shoe department and we will find a perfect replacement for you."

I asked the lady who told me her experience, "So, where do you buy all your shoes now?"

"Shoes?" she replied. "You mean, where do I buy *everything* now!"

That's what generous recovery looks like. Most people who hear this story are amazed at the generosity of the frontline clerk in giving away an expensive gift, two gifts, in this case. Others are impressed by the authority of a frontline clerk to make such decisions on the spot without a manager's permission. But the amazing part of this story is the fact that this clerk can go clear across the store to another department, under a different manager, who reports to a different vice president, and help herself to *their* inventory in order to satisfy *her* customer, whom they have never seen! She can also help herself to any cash register in the store and sell any item in any department. Can you imagine hospitals with this kind of empowerment and the invisible departmental walls it requires? Jack Welch calls it "borderlessness" at General Electric, a core principle on which he tried to build his management structure. If retail and manufacturing businesses are striving to tear down the structures that prevent teamwork and spontaneity, why not hospitals?

It can happen but it takes every manager being on the same page and supporting each other. It doesn't happen just because top management decrees it to happen. Gail Meadows, a laboratory director at a hospital in Florida, is an enthusiastic proponent of patient satisfaction and loyalty. Moved by the kind of empowerment that exists at places like Disney and Nordstrom, she went back to her staff and asked them, "What are some decisions I retain the power to make that keep you from taking care of problems immediately?"

One of the things they talked about was when they make a mistake that requires a patient to come back in for a repeat blood draw. If the patient complains, the phlebotomist can only apologize. If the patient seems to expect something taken off the bill for the double draw, the decision can be made only by the manager. The policy was changed immediately. Frontline lab staff had the authority to say, "Yes, of course, this will not cost you anything."

Gail told me what she had done. I congratulated her on giving up some of the authority to say Yes and decentralizing service recovery. But then I asked, "Doesn't writing off something only help the insurance company? It's the patient who is inconvenienced. What does the patient get out of this for the trouble caused by the lab's mistake?"

I went on to tell her about some focus groups conducted by Marriott. They had a service-recovery policy that would put the guest up in a more expensive room for free in a competitor's hotel if Marriott had to bump someone because another guest did not check out when expected. Marriott figured they lost about a thousand dollars every time this happened. Just to check how the policy was perceived by their guests, they conducted some focus groups of business people who had experienced it. What they learned was that although it cost Marriott a lot of money, it bought them very little loyalty from the guest. Here was the logic: "You sent me across town and gave me a free room in another hotel. But my employer is paying for my trip. So to pick up my tab doesn't benefit me personally; it only benefits my employer. I am the one who has to find transportation to and from my conference. I am the one who has been inconvenienced. There is nothing in your policy for me."

The facilitator representing Marriott then asked, "Would you rather we handed you $200 cash for your inconvenience and you paid your own way at the other hotel, instead of us picking up the expenses?" They all agreed they would. Notice what a win-win this turned out to be. Marriott went from spending $1,000 on service recovery to spending $200. And the customer is happier!

Gail went back to her staff and brought up what I had said. They joked about maybe sending a limousine like Nordstrom had done for a customer in another story I had told them. (Nordstrom in San Francisco had done this for a customer who had gotten back to her hotel and discovered the clerk had mismatched the shoes she bought.) They thought they were being facetious, but this triggered a useful notion. "What if we get home health to visit our patient and draw the blood for us when we goof up? They could also apologize and leave a gift certificate. We would have to pay them for the visit, but the patient would be very impressed and there would be a gift that benefits them instead of the insurance company."

In the end, Gail's staff decided to visit the patient's home themselves and leave a gift certificate after correcting their mistake by obtaining another blood sample.

Gail's leadership as a lab director also illustrates the truth that each department needs to have this conversation for themselves instead of waiting for administration to tell them what to do. A blanket policy for recovery sent down from on high can be directed only at the most trivial things. In the typical efforts I have seen, Gail's staff would never have assumed that administration meant for them to go over Gail's head and write off the bill, or send someone from home health to draw blood or give away gift certificates for a lab mistake without Gail's support. Only Gail, who has the power, can give that power away. And only department heads like Gail can inspire another department head to help out in their mutual goal of regaining the goodwill and loyalty of their patients when we let them down.

SOME SERVICE RECOVERY NEEDS TO BE STANDARDIZED.

At a recent Marriott stay, I received a fruit basket in my room when I was forced to move because of a problem that was the hotel's fault. What was interesting about this generous gift is that I did not complain about anything. Marriott automatically made the gesture when they asked me to move to another room.

Most hospitals with rudimentary service recovery policies only reward patients or families who complain. A sophisticated service recovery program would automatically trigger service recovery when something happens we know is frustrating to our patients whether they complain or not. For instance, being moved several times after being admitted is an inconvenience to a family. If the family gets angry and complains, most hospitals will send some flowers as recovery to the patient's room. But would they do the same if the family did not complain?

Like Gail in the lab recovery illustration, every unit dealing with patients would do well to make a list of frustrations and inconveniences that patients should not have to suffer, and devise a system of appropriate recoveries that are instituted automatically. In Gail's case, the recovery became automatic and was implemented by her staff on the spot without her involvement and without the patient needing to complain about it.

A HUDDLE CAN FACILITATE COMMUNICATION, RESPONSIBILITY AND TEAMWORK.

It is common practice at all the Disney facilities and resorts for cast members to meet with their manager every day in a "huddle" in their departments at the beginning of their shift. This is like its namesake in football, only it's more like the pre-game huddle teams have in the locker room before taking the field. Here the coach goes over, one more time, the plays they have practiced over and over. He fires up the team to do its best. He urges them on to attempt their greatest performance. He reiterates the obstacles and challenges that will likely face them on the field of play. He reminds them that character and good sportsmanship are important. He lets them know they are expected to do their organization and themselves proud. With a final cheer, the team charges out the door to do what they have been preparing to do. At Disney many managers use this effective technique to remind all cast members every day of how they are doing and what they could do better. They also have an opportunity during the huddle to ask questions. In an earlier chapter I described the daily huddle Debra Stacy has at the Knoxville Residence Inn with her staff.

It's interesting how often we talk about coaching as a leadership concept yet rarely do the things real coaches do almost religiously. Coaches can be all over the map in style and personality and even in coaching techniques, but all of them have pre-game huddles and pretty much do the same things in the huddle. Imagine a great coach giving one pep talk at the beginning of the season, scheduling daily practices, and then letting the team just show up for each game on time and start playing when the referee blows his whistle! If the huddle is so important in athletic team performance, why isn't it standard practice in organizations like hospitals where teamwork is just as crucial?

Nurses have always had their form of the huddle at change-of-shift time. They call it "giving report." It's imperative in nursing for continuity of patient care. But it's rarely used to inspire the staff or communicate what is going on in the emergency department or other areas of the hospital. Most departments would benefit from a huddle at the beginning of every shift.

At some hospitals where I have been, they have instituted a daily administrative huddle of key department heads or their assistants around eight o'clock in the morning. They have discovered it to be a great way to share information, ask for help, and work together between departments to solve problems and shorten the decision-making cycle. First they get a report from the night supervisor. Then they go over the "state of the house": how many patients, what serious cases are of special concern, how well staffed they are, how backed up the emergency department is, what a physician is concerned about, who is feeling overwhelmed, how they can help each other in stressful circumstances, who is going to be off next week, etc. Where department heads or their assistants have been doing this, they find it saves much more time than it takes each day. They are able to take care of many things immediately, face-to-face, instead of playing telephone tag or stopping to send e-mails and waiting for answers.

One of the surprising things I have taken from all the focus groups I have conducted through the years with managers and supervisors is that any department can be the star example of internal service and responsiveness. A department that shines in one hospital will be the department that creates the most frustration in another. One place will have nothing but scorn for pharmacy or human resources or engineering or housekeeping or food service or administration. Then at another place they will rave about how outstanding one of these same departments is at their facility.

For instance, in one hospital virtually all the focus groups talked about how frustrating it was to deal with engineering. They were not responsive. You never knew when they would show up. They sent two guys to do little jobs that needed only one. They never cleaned up after themselves. If you complained, they were rude and made you feel as if your requests would go to the bottom of the list. Their supervisor was never available to go over major plans in renovation and began projects without consulting the people who worked in the areas where changes were being made.

In contrast another hospital sang the praises of their engineering staff. They were courteous and responsive. They could be depended on to be on time and get the work done efficiently. They were easy to work with and friendly to everybody. After hearing these accolades, I stopped one of the engineering staff in the hallway and told him about what I was hearing about his department. I asked him what they do that makes them so appreciated. He was at a loss to say. In probing, however, I discovered that anybody is willing to take a work order. You can call the department or stop one of the workers in the hall and make a request. That person will see to it that the request gets handled properly. Jobs are rarely assigned by a supervisor. Instead, they meet in a huddle every morning with their supervisor to discuss and prioritize the jobs together. Assignments are more or less volunteered for. Everyone feels responsible for all the work instead of just for what the supervisor assigns.

In the 1980s, British Airways commissioned a widely publicized study to determine what matters most to frequent flyers. What was most surprising to management was how important a characteristic called *spontaneity* was in customer loyalty. Spontaneity was described as *the ability of frontline employees to solve problems spontaneously on the spot.*

We don't need to duplicate this study in other service industries to believe how important it is for the people who deal with customers to be able to make decisions that solve problems and give good service immediately.

---

1. W. Steven Brown, *13 Fatal Errors Managers Make and How You Can Avoid Them* (New York: Berkley Books, 1985), p. 10.
2. Peter M. Senge, "Leading Learning Organizations: The Bold, the Powerful, and the Invisible," in Frances Hesselbein, Marshall Goldsmith, and Richard Beckhard, eds., *The Leader of the Future: New Visions, Strategies, and Practices for the Next Era* (San Francisco: Jossey-Bass Publishers, 1996), pp. 42-44.

Chapter

6
Change the Concept of Work from Service to Theater

Everyone expects Disney to regard entertainment work as theater. After all, they are in the entertainment business. They are trying to create an escape from reality. When guests enter the world of Disney, they enter a make-believe world of fantasy and fun. But a hospital is about as real as life can get and as far from most people's fantasy of fun as anyone can imagine. Here, where patients are hurting, sad, anxious, and depressed, entertainment is not what they are looking for. Would Disney really define work as theater if they ran your hospital? Absolutely. And here's why: Disney World is not a service; it's an experience. So are movies and plays. Hospitalization is not a service either; it's an experience. Disney World provides a stage to facilitate the experience of fun. Hospitalization provides a stage to facilitate the experience of healing. For both Disney and hospitals, it is more accurate to describe their business as *providing a transforming dramatic experience* than delivering a service. Not all drama is meant to be fun. But all successful drama is a transforming experience.

Using the word "service" to describe hospital work has never felt quite right, especially to bedside caregivers. Improving patient care by calling it service excellence may have been the best we could come up with in the last two decades, but it misses something that is hard to put your finger on until you understand Disney's business model, which focuses on how to improve the guest's experience instead of how to provide better service. In fact I have found that the best way to revitalize many stalled service-excellence initiatives in hospitals is to make this shift in emphasis from the caregiver's service to the patient's experience. Just changing the language of service and courtesy to one that highlights experience and theater is refreshing and often energizing.

WE NEED TO SHIFT THE SERVICE-EXCELLENCE PARADIGM.

Hospital work is theater whether we call it that or not. In this context the word "theater" is not a metaphor. Scores of management metaphors abound—soaring with eagles, leading like geese, flying with the buffalo, herding cats, swimming with sharks, dancing with elephants, training whales, moving with the cheese—to name a few. But even though each of these spotlights a particular aspect of leadership, none is a comprehensive model. Hospital work is not *like* theater; it *is* theater. It is a business model, every bit as differentiated from services as services are differentiated from goods.

For a comprehensive analysis of and detailed process for applying the power of the theater business model in the latest evolution to gain and keep customers, read *The Experience Economy*, by B. Joseph Pine II and James H. Gilmore. They describe four ascending levels of economic offering: commodities, goods, services, and experiences. With each offering, value and profits increase exponentially. Take coffee for example. As a commodity, it goes for about 2 cents a cup. Packaging it and selling it as goods, jumps the price to 20 cents a cup. Sell it as a service in a coffee shop, and it's worth about a dollar. However, include that cup of coffee as part of an experience staged with all the ambience of an exclusive restaurant or the stimulation of a bookstore that encourages you to "have a cup of coffee with your favorite author," and consumers will gladly pay $2 to $5. As the authors state:

Experiences are a fourth economic offering, as distinct from services as services are from goods, but one that has until now gone largely unrecognized. Experiences have always been around, but consumers, businesses, and economists lumped them into the service sector along with such uneventful activities as dry cleaning, auto repair, wholesale distribution, and telephone access...

But this doesn't mean that experiences rely exclusively on entertainment; entertainment is only one aspect of an experience. Rather, companies stage an experience whenever they *engage* customers, connecting with them in a personal, memorable way.

While commodities are fungible, goods tangible, and services intangible, experiences are memorable...

All prior economic offerings remain at arms-length, outside the buyer, while experiences are inherently personal. They actually occur within any individual who has been engaged on an emotional, physical, intellectual, or even spiritual level. The result? No two people can have the same experience—period. Each experience derives from the interaction between the staged event and the individual's prior state of mind and being.[1]

Can there be any question where a hospital fits along this continuum? To paraphrase the authors' definition: *Hospitals are providing experiences that engage patients on an emotional, physical, intellectual, and, yes, spiritual level*, whether the patients frame it as such in their minds or not. Hospital guests do not talk about the services they received. They talk about the experiences they had. Poor service is the surest way to turn a service into a bad experience, remembered and talked about for years.

When hospital personnel view their work as engaging the patient in a memorable experience, instead of just trying to give "excellent service," the shift is one of substance, a true paradigm shift. And no business provides better proof of the value of this shift than Disney, where, according to Pine and Gilmore, the idea originated and is now being emulated by bookstores (Barnes and Noble, Borders), airlines

(Southwest), restaurants (Chucky Cheese, McDonald's), car dealers (Saturn, Lexus), and retail stores (Brookstone, Sharper Image) and a host of other businesses.

In our own industry look at the success and recognition attained by the hospitals that have adopted variations of the Planetree model, where every aspect of the patient's and family's interactions and accommodations have been carefully scripted and staged to provide a memorable, total experience. They exemplify the conceptual shift that the Disney business model brings to a hospital, the shift from providing services to staging experiences.

WALKING THE TALK IMPLIES A STAGE.

When we use phrases like "walk the talk" or "role-modeling" we are using theatrical terms. They underscore the fact that people are watching and that what they see influences their beliefs and behavior. Employees who talk about leaders walking the talk or role-modeling behaviors are telling us that their leaders are also on stage, and as an audience, employees are just as engaged and influenced as customers by what they hear and see.

Whether the performer is aware of it or not, he or she is always communicating. The subtle expressions of tone of voice, facial expression, and body language may not be under the control of conscious thought, but they can still convey powerful and dramatic messages. The goal of making hospital work into theater is to engage all the guest's senses, in an experience in which each performing member of the cast conveys a message congruent with conscious intentions that have been discussed, internalized, and rehearsed by the director, the playwright, and the team of performers and stagehands. (Notice how naturally theatrical terms fit the hospital drama.)

In fact we use many phrases already in hospital parlance that are theatrical in origin or nature:

Performance	Star performers	Directing
Setting	Engaging	Scripting
Rapport	Relating	Roles
Talent		

IT STARTS WITH A GOOD SCRIPT
WHICH IS MORE THAN DIALOGUE.

Probably the most popular textbook for aspiring directors to study is Harold Clurman's, *On Directing*. Notice how his definition of theater resonates with Pine and Gilmore's "experience economy" and work as theater: "Theatre is a particular mode of expression through which a community realizes itself. The audience is the theatre's wellspring, its leading actor. This is not a metaphor; it is a historical fact."[2]

"Choose a good script," he often admonishes his students, "cast good actors–and you'll all be good directors."[3] The Disney organization would agree. Aspiring directors of hospital work processes would be well served by the same admonition.

A common practice in hospitals today is "scripting" which, to most managers, means simply writing out what employees are supposed to say in repetitive situations. Not so in theater. In theater the script is much more than just the words actors are supposed to say. A script maps out the entire experience, scene by scene. Everything that contributes to the desired outcome of the drama is in the script. It specifies the details and cues needed to carry out the intentions of every scene. It usually includes time frames, transitions between scenes, actions, set decoration, props, casting notes, actor's appearance, staging details, and even subtext (what's going on beneath the surface in the actor's mind). Before it is produced, it is also shaped by the director's extensive notes about the story, the spine (driving force behind actions and intentions), the atmosphere, the movement between characters, and a host of nuances not in the original script.

At Disney scripts are a collaborative effort, not the work of one playwright. Walt Disney is credited with the "storyboard" method of developing a plot and a script through collective brainstorming. Everyone can contribute to the shaping of the story because the storyboard is set up where all can see it and add their ideas on index cards. Since the cards are pinned to a corkboard-like surface, they can be freely moved, deleted, or expanded with details. Once the storyline is developed, complete with scenes and artistic cues, the staff begins the actual work of staging the experience for the audience within the constraints of the budget, medium, and tools they are using.

Script development, then, is really akin to designing and mapping clinical processes. Desired outcomes (experiences) determine what events (scenes) need to take place in what settings (stage) with what people (performers). Within each scene careful attention is paid to everything that is done to move the patient's experience along to a successful conclusion. Process improvement teams often use Disney's storyboard technique to brainstorm the ideal process and ways in which a process can be improved. Diagnostic methods are used to measure and track key activities to make sure improvement is taking place. As in a good drama, the more attention is paid to the details of the process, the more predictable and effective the outcome will be.

So what does the concept of scripting contribute to the activity of process mapping or planning? Several important things:

1. It focuses on much more than just the mechanical process steps, clinical outcomes, or efficiency, as most process improvement teams do. It takes in the totality of the experience and the patient's emotional (and spiritual) needs as well. In fact, a script puts the patient's emotional experience and human interactions at the heart of the healing process, not as an add-on.

2. It is the concrete expression of vision. Most hospitals express their vision in terms of desired outcomes, but a script ensures that the vision, not just the work, is scripted in detail, making sure each scene and each encounter contributes to that vision.

3. It describes the role and character that a person must play for the patient to experience healing at all levels, not just the physical. It includes how people are expected to relate to each other and to the patient in each scene. Scripts make clear what is expected in an actor's performance, what must be conveyed and what is not conveyed, regardless of how the performer feels.

It's too bad many hospitals have gotten the idea of scripting as a rote adherence to dialogue written by a committee. Workers often, and rightly, feel it is condescending to tell them to say "please" and "thank you" and other obvious phrases that get put into the scripts everyone is supposed to use.

Do you remember the first time you flew on Southwest Airlines? Whatever you were doing at the time, I'll bet you dropped it and looked

up in astonishment when the flight attendant started the s
the beginning of the flight. We have all become accustome
repetition of the safety script. Suddenly, something we h
tune out for its monotony was entertaining and sounded spontaneous.
After hearing many of these, I now know that most of the material is
spontaneous. No two speakers give it exactly alike. And all of them
seem to be having fun with something that appears to bore attendants
on other airlines. Meanwhile, as an audience, I am engaged and their
required spiel becomes a memorable experience.

At Disney's Wilderness Lodge I observed the valet cast members
greeting cars as they drove up to check into the resort. I expected to
hear each valet greet each car in the same way, even if it was his own
way, but they didn't. In fact they all had slightly different greetings and
they seemed to have different ways of relating to the new guests. So I
went to their supervisor and asked if they had a script for the valets. He
said, "Well, it's not exactly a script. What we do is teach them to do four
things: (1) Give a great big over-the-top welcome (with a big smile, of
course) to the Wilderness Lodge. (2) Notice the license plate and say
something about their state, or city, or the weather back home. (3)
Wave and speak immediately through the window to any children.
And, (4) notice anything interesting, like a bumper sticker, sports decal,
or custom paint job, and comment on it." The supervisor went on to
tell me that new cast members work with the best valets the first few
days on the job and practice doing these four things with a lot of
personality. The point is they are instructed to be alert to cues from the
guests and respond to them. All this before they even do the job of
helping with the luggage.

Now is that a script? Yes, it is. It's not rote dialogue but it is still a
script. There is an adherence to certain engagement and courtesy
guidelines, but the actual words are the person's own. Spontaneity is
part of the script to keep the dialogue natural.

Most movie directors will say that adhering to the *intent* of a scene
is much more important than adhering to the actual *words* in the script.
Once actors are in tune with the purpose of the scene and the desired
response from the audience, they are often free to use their own words
and actions. The script does not change, but the words may.

.ien one realizes that hospital work is theater because it is staging an experience, one can understand how important the script is. I believe hospital scripts should teach all hospital workers how to enter a hospital room and engage the patient. Like valets at the Wilderness Lodge, they should: (1) Greet the patient by name and introduce themselves with a cheerful greeting. (2) Comment on anything special in the room like flowers or pictures of family. (3) Meet any other people that are in the room. (4) Ask if there is anything else they need or need explained. (5) Empathize with any expressions of feeling. (6) Ask how they want the door left (open, closed, or partially open). (7) Remember conversations from each day to build on over the duration of the patient's stay. And, yes, all this *before* the task they came to perform.

Personally I like Walt Disney's approach to script writing. Hospital units or departments should brainstorm each moment of truth with three columns: *What We Do, what the guest needs to know and feel,* and *What We Say* to engage our guests in a memorable way.

This is not a rote string of words to be delivered verbatim. But neither is it allowing hospital workers simply to wing it with no training or practice, so that some appear friendly and helpful and others barely say a word that engages the patient. Remember, the nurse is staging an experience, not delivering a service. So is the person who delivers the food tray. So is the physical therapist. So is the transporter. Direct and coach them all that they are there to create a memorable experience in each scene with the patient. Then get them to collaborate by helping to develop the scripts and demonstrating how they do it.

CONSISTENCY IS A HALLMARK OF GREAT PERFORMANCES.

One of the marks of a world-class organization is its ability to repeat a performance over and over with the same consistency. Performers who cannot deliver the same powerful show or recital day in and day out on the stage, are quickly let go. Great stage actors have learned uncompromising self-discipline in addition to their talent. They know that each performance must be just as good as the last. There is no for moodiness or letting how they feel at the moment interfere eir total commitment to the script, the audience, the other cast members, and the director. Actors are inspired by stories of their favorite actors who went "on with the show" in spite of personal tragedy, debilitating stage fright, and painful physical ailments. There must never be a bad day or a lousy show. And if there is, one has not lived up to his or her commitment as an actor.

In my experience with attempts to improve the interpersonal skills of the staff at hospitals, those who demonstrate outstanding performances day in and day out, rarely get praised for it. We like to single out those who did something "above and beyond" to please a guest, but we often take for granted the consistent repetition of desired behaviors by dependable performers. Like great actors they make it look easy every day of the week. They deliver with the same freshness, power, and energy on their thousandth performance as they did on their first.

By introducing theater language into our hospital work, we can make concepts like "the show must go on" and "for every guest, this is their first time" take an elevated place in our thinking. By recognizing and appreciating our most consistent performers, we place value on repetitious behaviors that engage the patient and win their love and loyalty.

CASTING GOOD ACTORS HELPS MAKE A GOOD DIRECTOR.

The opening of Disneyland in Anaheim on a hot day in July 1955 was a disaster. Thousands of counterfeit tickets were sold. The crowds were far bigger than anyone expected. Part of the park was not working. According to Bob Thomas, Walt Disney's official biographer, "Every street within a ten-mile radius of the park was clogged with automobiles...Rides broke down...Restaurants and refreshment stands ran out of food and drink. A gas leak was detected in Fantasyland, and the entire area was closed to the public. Tempers flared as the sun grew hotter...the Mark Twain steamboat with its decks awash because of too many passengers...parents tossing small children over the heads of the crowd to gain rides on the King Arthur Carousel." Ever afterward Walt referred to opening day as "Black Sunday."[4]

Walt Disney learned many hard lessons from that day, but one of them was the absolute necessity to have control over the behavior of every single employee. An outside agency had provided the security personnel, and the complaints about their conduct convinced him that every security person who ever works at Disneyland must work for Disney and have a talent for handling people in a gracious, friendly manner. No member of the cast can be out of step with the purpose of the company, which in Disney's words is "to make people happy."

Many years ago I had the opportunity to go through a simulation exercise at Disney in Orlando. Each table of participants, except one table in the middle, was instructed to get acquainted with each other and then choose one member to apply for the job of security officer. We were allowed to make up a fictitious resume for the individual. At my table we did our task with relish and picked the most imposing looking man to be our candidate.

The table in the center of the room was asked to create a job description for a security officer for Disney World and then interview the various candidates for three minutes. Then they were to choose one candidate for the job and explain why to the entire group.

We were sure our big guy would win, but he didn't. The person chosen was a pleasant woman with a lovely smile. In the discussion that followed we saw that our table was biased by our own image of a security officer. The table that won looked at it from the point of view of the *experience* guests expected to have at Disney. They chose a person who fit the character they needed to play a role in a production that was designed "to make people happy." The casting group had described just such a person at their table before doing the brief interviews. When you know what you want, it doesn't take long to make a decision on a person's fit with the organization. In Jim Collin's book, *Built to Last*, he quotes Walt Disney on casting for a role instead of a job.

> The first year I leased out the parking concession, brought in the usual security guards–things like that. But I soon realized my mistake. I couldn't have outside help and still get over my idea of hospitality. So now we recruit and train every one of our employees. I tell the security officers, for instance, that they are

never to consider themselves cops. They are there
people.[5]

One of the serious detractors for hospital work as theater is .
constant turnover in staff and the significant use of agency nurses. Walt
Disney would be the first to say this is a recipe for inconsistent and poor
performance. He is purported to have said, "Casting means finding the
best people and keeping them so they can practice together and become
a proficient ensemble." (Manual at Disney University)

AUDITION FOR TALENT RATHER THAN SKILLS TO PERFORM ROLES RATHER THAN JOBS.

One of the most desirable consequences of using the theater model is
in the way it elevates work by hiring on the basis of the talent needed
to engage the audience (customer) and the vital role they play in that,
rather than the skills needed to do a particular job, like drawing blood
or registering patients or serving food.

Whenever I have a small audience of frontline employees, I ask
participants to introduce themselves and tell me what their role is in
the hospital. Almost without exception each person mentions the
department and then describes his or her work. If I probe with
"And how do you go about doing that?" they usually describe the
specific tasks they perform.

For example, somebody says, "I work in registration."

I ask, "What does that mean?"

She might say, "It means I register the patient. You know, I get their
age and address, their insurance information, who their doctor is, why
they are being admitted, things like that. And I assign them a number
and print out a wrist band for them."

Next I might ask, "Why did they pick you for this role?" I suspect
she would say, "I don't know," or that she had some computer skills.
Who would ever think to say, "They hired me because I make a great
first impression"? Or "Because I am super friendly and helpful"?

Why don't employees say that? Because nobody stressed the role
they play in providing the best possible experience for the patient. In

service paradigm only the service (entering data in the computer) and common courtesy gets evaluated as performance.

This person, like everyone else, has assumed the word "role" means her job. However, if she had been hired in an experience/theater paradigm as they do at Disney, she would have known that her role is bigger than her job. Her director (manager, supervisor) who worked from a script (ideal process) would have made it clear that her primary role is to play a character who engages the patient in a memorable experience. And as the first contact person in the hospital, this role has a major impact—first impression—on the patient. She would certainly have to learn the mechanics of the computer and the codes for various insurance companies, but she would know that whoever hired her thought she had the talent to play the role of first contact with the patient and the patient's family. Her character's role, according to a complete script, is to make guests feel welcome, cared about, and reassured. It is her role to get them off to a friendly start. It is her role to engender trust in the healthcare team. It is her role to help them find their way around an unfamiliar place. Finally, and most importantly, it is her role that defines the talent she needs. This means her director's primary concern is to look for and hire that talent. Real talent, like a great welcoming persona, cannot be taught, but computer skills and insurance codes can.

Once the director has hired for the welcoming talent called for in the script, the role must be defined to capitalize on that talent. Orientation and rehearsal should emphasize the personal requirements for the role. Constant praise and little tune-ups are also needed to reinforce the person's role, not just the tasks that the person does. In our focus on efficiency and accuracy, it is easy to lose sight of this without continuous reminders.

Each director in the hospital has an obligation to go through the same process of auditioning for the talent required in every role, which is greater than the skills needed in the task. Imagine a director of housekeeping telling a new employee, "I need you to play a housekeeper who loves patients. Can you do that? I need you to get into your friendliest character every time you step onto the floor (stage), and no matter how you are feeling that day, your performance will be the same: friendly, cheerful, helpful, and sympathetic. Can you Because if you can't I will find someone who can. Anyone can clean a room, but not everyone is suited to play the role that I am asking you to play every day when you come to work. I need someone in your position who has the talent to engage our patients and guests in a memorable way while you go about your work, and I hope it will be you."

One of the most successful restaurants in the world is California Grill at the top of Disney's Contemporary Resort. The manager was George Miliotes. His staff was an amazing ensemble of cast members that regularly received tips of 30 percent. He told a group of us his amazingly simple criteria for hiring. "We have a huge list of applicants. Every waiter and waitress in town wants to work here. In the beginning my chef and I made a list of about 20 attributes we were looking for. But in the end, I guess, I pretty much look for just two things. Is this person happy and is this person smart? If you are smart, we can teach you anything. If you are happy, I know you will make the customers happy." Even in a prestigious restaurant, experience and skill were secondary to talent.

I asked him what he asked when auditioning new talent. He said, "I have a normal conversation with the person, as a customer does. I ask easy things like what he or she likes to do most, what's fun, etc. One of my favorite questions is 'Why do you want to work here?' If they say anything about the money or how it will look on their resume, I probably pass on them. What I want to hear them talk about is how much they love serving people, making them happy, and working with a group of great cast members to provide an unforgettable evening for our guests—things like that."

Not bad questions, I might add, for auditioning performers in healthcare. One night I overheard my wife on the phone checking a reference for someone who had applied to fill a vacancy in nursing management. I was surprised to hear her say, "Yes, but is she fun? You know, F-U-N. Is she any fun?"

When she ended the conversation I asked in mock surprise, "Fun? Since when is that a requirement to be a nurse manager?"

"Well, what do you call it when you're always glad to see someone. Someone who lights up everybody's day. A manager who everybody hugs when she gets back from vacation? A person who makes people around her feel happy?"

"I guess I have always called that a 'positive attitude,' " I said.

"Well, how weak is that!" she exclaimed. "Everyone has a so-called positive attitude, but not everybody is fun. I need a nursing team who like each other and have fun together. Heaven knows their jobs are hard enough without having to deal with moody managers. A positive attitude is not good enough."

It reminded me of George Miliotes looking for a happy person.

Terry Barter, the director of rehabilitation and sports medicine at Florida Hospital, whose staff had made a great impression on me, told me that he looked for the talents of service-mindedness and team spirit when interviewing new physical therapists. I asked him how he screens for that in a job interview (audition).

"I think you have to give the person a scenario and see how he would handle it," he said. "For instance, one of the scenarios I sometimes give is this: 'You get to a patient's room on time for your physical therapy appointment, but the patient is not ready because he has soiled his sheets and needs cleaning up. What would you do?' "

"If the person says, 'I would go tell the nurse,' I would then ask, 'What if the nurse says she can't get to it right now?' "

"If the person says he would reschedule, or go early to his next appointment and come back later, I probably wouldn't hire him. What I am looking for is a person who will say, 'I'd clean up the patient myself.' And if he never mentions trying to get the nurse, that's even better. It's a lot easier to hire a person who will automatically pitch in on unpleasant tasks than it is to require someone to do it whose mindset is 'that's not my job.' It's not easy, and I don't bat a thousand in selecting perfect people, but I have to keep trying and telling people what's most important and thanking them when they come through."

WE SHOULD TEACH ACTING SKILLS INSTEAD OF BODY LANGUAGE.

Acting is not pretending. This is a common misunderstanding that we have about the notion of acting. Surely, to a nurse, the idea of pretending to care when you don't would be offensive. Up until this point I have used the word "performance" because it is a common word in our hospital vocabulary and roughly means the same thing. Still I cannot leave this chapter on using theater vocabulary without addressing this misconception about acting, the heart of theater.

Several years ago I thought it would be fun to sign up for an actor's workshop. It met once a week in the evening. I remember how hard it was to please our acting coach. The problem was being "real." When we practiced our scenes in front of her, she would say, "I could see you acting." So in acting class, "acting" was a bad word! We spent much more time learning how to "come from a real place," as she called it, than in learning our lines or anything else. She taught us that we cannot act sad. We have to really be sad. Acting (pretending) is something easily perceived. You can't fake it. The audience can tell, and will call it bad acting.

So how do you come from a real place? We learned that it is through imagination. We spent hours searching our lives for when we had experienced intense emotions: anger, humiliation, shame, grief, humor, joy, sensuality, playfulness, hatred, betrayal. These memories were called "sensory choices" and became the focus of our thoughts when saying our lines. We were taught to imagine our sensory choice when the scene called for a certain emotion and to stay fixated on it in our minds through the scene, despite all the distractions of props, actors, cameras, and lights.

We learned the power of our choices in making nonverbal cues congruent with the feelings needed in a scene by sharing them with the group. For instance one evening we sat around in a circle and the teacher had each of us describe the saddest scene in our lives. We were not to tell anything about what led up to the scene or what followed the scene. We were just to describe it vividly. That was all.

I thought about the saddest time of my life and said something like this: "I am in a beautiful place on a beautiful day. The sun is shining. There are long shadows from the trees on my left. In front of me . . ."

Suddenly I felt my eyes filling with tears. I stared at the floor. What I had just said seemed so incongruous with the emotions that had instantly welled up inside of me. I continued. "In front of me there is a casket waiting to be lowered into the ground. My little daughter, only five years old, is standing there in a pink and white dress. She is holding a flower in her tiny hand. Nearby, her little brother and others are watching."

My voice broke and the tears brimmed over their restraints. "She throws the flower on the casket," I choked, "and then I hear a forlorn little voice ask, 'Is mommy really in there?' "

When I gained enough composure to look up, the entire group, which had bonded over the weeks we had spent in that workshop sharing together, had tears in their eyes too.

My sensory imagination made me come from a real place. But the amazing thing is that *their* imagination put them in the same place with me. Nobody was acting. My pain and their empathy were real. No wonder patients who are dealt some of life's cruelest blows can experience healing when they are with fellow sufferers in a therapy group who will wrap them in a blanket of compassion and empathy. Through imagination, however, we can give that blessing to anyone. Any actor who tries to play a serious scene by pretending would probably be turned out of the play and labeled a poor actor. The reason for this is that if there is one thing that defines an actor's talent, it is his or her ability to be real in a scene. If actors are rich in a gift, it is the gift of being in touch with all parts of their personalities and their feelings through imagination. In psychological terms we would say that they have the capacity, on demand, to be emotionally available.

If a nurse holds the hand of a weeping patient and even sheds a tear, we would not insult her by accusing her of pretending. She was being real with the patient by allowing herself to be open to the patient's feelings. She was also acting, in the finest sense of the word. The patient's pain was not happening to her, but through the nurse's own imagination (acting), the patient experiences empathy and understanding—two of nature's greatest healing gifts.

If compassion is so important in hospitals, managers need to understand it and treat it as a talent that needs to be recruited, developed, and role modeled. Compassion has to come from a real place, as they say in acting, or it will be perceived as an act. Eric Morris is one of the most renowned acting coaches in the world. He served as chairman of the director's unit of the Actor's Studio and now runs the Eric Morris Actors Workshop in Los Angeles, where many famous actors go to rediscover their talent and hone their skills. His books on acting are considered essential reading by aspiring actors. The title of his latest book is *No Acting Please—A Revolutionary Approach to Acting and Living*. The title emphasizes the truth that acting is not pretending. And if we are not pretending, we are being real, which means we are really living. The ability to be real and in touch with our own real feelings and the feelings of those around us can enrich our lives and enhance our relationships. It is not an exaggeration to say that being real is the secret to acting and living. As Eric Morris says in the opening paragraph of his book:

> Acting is the art of creating genuine realities on a stage. No matter what the material, the actor's fundamental question is: "What is the reality and how can I make it real to *me*?" In this kind of training the actor discovers himself fully both on the stage and off, since the exercises in this book repeatedly demand an integration of living and acting. It is a way of life, not just a way of work.[6]

And, we might add, so is nursing. To paraphrase Eric Morris, Nursing is the art of creating genuine realities on the sterile, impersonal stage of a hospital room. No matter what the task (read "scene"), the nurse's fundamental question is: "What is the reality of this patient's experience, and how can I make it real to me?"

Theater changes our focus from our task to the patient's experience. Bud Owens, a director of emergency services, tells about the final days of his beloved "granny," who had moved into his home when he was five years old after the death of his grandfather. She had helped to raise him and he loved her very much. Even though he was a little kid for his age, she always called him Big Boy. During her last hospitalization she lapsed into a coma. Her family stood around her bed for hours in her intensive care room, hoping for a glimmer of awareness before she died.

When the charge nurse discovered how long they had been in the patient's room she scolded them for not following the rules and ushered them down the hall to the chapel. The chaplain visited the family there, and when they told him about the incident, he took it upon himself to escort the family back to the intensive care unit where they were able to continue their vigil. Bud says that he will always be grateful to that chaplain because his grandmother stirred, opened her eyes and looked right at him. "Is that you, Big Boy?" she asked. "I love you, Big Boy." Those were her last words.

"I can't tell you how much that moment meant to me," Bud recalls. "Yet I still get angry when I think how close we came to missing it because of that charge nurse."

In a similar vein, Ellen Liston, head of marketing at Children's Hospital in Knoxville, told me about the tragic loss of her brother-in-law, Jason, who was barely 30 when he died of complications from brain tumors. Although he fought the debilitating symptoms for more than a year, he finally succumbed, and on a July weekend he lay dying as his young wife, two daughters, parents, extended family members, and friends said their good-byes in his hospital room.

Ellen says, "Around 11 P.M. that evening, Jason's breathing became very labored and shallow, and none of us would even leave his bedside. Wendy, Jason's wife, looked at all of us and said that she wished it wasn't so late because she wished she could call a lady from their church to come again and sing for Jason. The lady had come earlier in the week and sung some of Jason's favorite hymns, and both Wendy and Jason seemed to draw great comfort from both the message of the songs and their friend's voice. In what seemed like only seconds later, a nurse named Cathy came in the room to check on Jason. I don't know if she heard Wendy talking or if God truly sent her in to help us, but there she was. She had actually just gone off duty, but she wanted to check on Jason. Cathy asked us what kind of music Jason liked, and we told her gospel music. She asked if he had any favorite songs, and my sister-in-law mentioned a few songs. Then Cathy just began to sing 'I'll Fly Away' and 'Amazing Grace.' I think she sang two other songs, but none of us can agree on what those songs were. What all of us did agree on is that we felt like an angel had been sent to take care of Jason and minister to our souls. We all just stood there listening, smiling at the beauty of the songs' messages while tears streamed down our cheeks. It was painful and joyous at the same time but gave each of us great peace because we felt that God had truly sent an angel to be with us in Jason's final hours."

These are two stories about the painful lingering moments in a loved one's life on the clinical stage of a hospital room. Two nurses going about their work—yet what a difference in the experience for the family! One made the family feel as if they were intruding on her busy world. The other, already checked out for the day, entered into the grieving experience with the family and, like an angel sent from God, shared herself in an unforgettable way.

GET ACQUAINTED WITH THE PATIENT'S PERSONAL STORY.

In theater the audience watches a performance that engages them in someone else's story. Obviously we have a different frame of reference for the theater of bedside care. For us the audience and the story are largely the same thing. Just as an actor must get into the mind, heart, and soul of a character through empathy, nurses have the opportunity to create a powerful healing experience by doing the same thing.

A nurse who worked in an Alzheimer's unit told me that during her first week on the job, her director took her by the hand as said, "Come with me, I want to show you something." She led her into a resident's room and pointed to some momentoes the family had placed in the room.

"This is a picture of Mary's family," she said. "Here's her wedding picture. And over here is Mary with her two daughters. This one is a violinist who plays with the Orlando symphyony, and I understand this one teaches French literature at some college. Did you know that Mary speaks fluent French? Her father fought in the war and married a French girl. He stayed there for many years to help her family. That's why Mary has these French books over here."

They went into all twelve of the resident rooms and the director repeated the process, telling the nurse about each resident. "I will never forget how that tour changed my attitude towards my patients," she told me. "They became real people to me instead of just patients. I saw them for who they were instead of what they had become. It made me more caring and empathetic because I felt I knew each one personally."

Something that can help enrich the caregiver's engagement with the patient, and generate empathy, is getting acquainted with the patient's personal story. Hospitals that have adopted a systematic way of doing this report a deeper connection for both caregivers and patients. During the initial process of admitting a patient, a "storyteller" interviews the patient to learn pertinent personal details about their lives that humanize them. The patient's story is printed and attached to the beginning of the patient's chart. Every caregiver who must care for the patient is expected to read the one-page document just as they read the other information on the chart. This helps doctors, nurses, and other clinicians to interact on a personal level with the patient. It also helps the caregiver as actor to enter into the patient's experience through imagination, which is the subject of the next chapter of this book.

It is acting, then (which means *no acting, please*), that can change a job into a calling. It can enable us to live life deeply, empathetically, and with intention. It connects us with the deepest parts of ourselves and the human condition. If all the world is a stage, then acting, allowing ourselves to be touched by the experiences of others, is the means by which the world can become connected in understanding and love

---

1. B. Joseph Pine II and James H. Gilmore, *The Experience Economy: Work Is Theater & Every Business a Stage* (Boston: Harvard Business School Press, 1999), pp. 2-12.

2. Harold Clurman, *On Directing* (New York: Simon & Schuster, 1997), p. 155.

3. Ibid., p. 64.

4. Bob Thomas, *Walt Disney, An American Original*, (New York: Simon and Schuster, 1976), p.272.

5. James C. Collins and Jerry I. Porras, *Built to Last* (New York: HarperCollins Publishers, Inc.), p. 131.

6. Eric Morris and Joan Hotchkis, *No Acting Please: "Beyond the Method" A Revolutionary Approach to Acting and Living* (Los Angeles: Ermor Enterprises Publishing, 1995), p. 1.

CHAPTER 7 HARNESS THE MOTIVATING POWER OF IMAGINATION

In a book about Disney, you would expect a lot about imagination. We could summon a thousand instances of inventions, films, merchandise, entertainment, and experiences born in the imagination of creative minds. Creative thinking is a valuable asset to any organization, and we need to make every effort to encourage its use in solving problems and improving systems. But creative imagination is not what this chapter is about. It's about *motivational* imagination and it builds on the acting theme developed in the last chapter.

During my first day in Disney Traditions, our instructor used imagination to motivate us. "Imagine some good friends whom you have not seen for a long time but would love to see," he said. "You just found out that they will be here on Friday to spend the weekend with you. What will you do to get ready for their visit?"

We made a list. Clean the bathrooms and hang up clean towels. Change the sheets on the bed. Vacuum the carpets. Stock up on special food and drinks we think they will like. Mow the lawn. Wash the cars. The list went on.

Then he asked us to make another list. "What are some things you would do or refrain from doing while they are here if you want them to have a good time and come back again?"

ch table we made a second list. Cater to them. Ask them what
ited to do and do it with them. Let them use the bathroom first.
em good food and be eager to refill their glasses. Be polite and
friendly. Respect their privacy. Be up before they are so we can greet
them in the morning. Ask them if they're having a good time. Smile and
be cheerful around them. Dress nicely. Don't pick your nose. Say please
and thank you and excuse me. Play the kind of music we know they
like. Don't air the family's personal problems in front of them. Put their
needs first. The lists varied, but these were the kinds of thoughts that
were expressed.

Then our instructor pointed to the combined list of our answers on
his flip chart. "We all know how to treat a guest in our home, don't we?
It's no different at Disney. We are hosts, every one of us. Our customers
are called guests. Please treat them as you would if you knew each one
of them personally and liked them. Treat them as you would if they
were staying in your own home. And do it every day, all the time. Help
us keep our promise to them that we are here to make them happy—
just as you would make your own guests happy."

This is using imagination for motivation, not creativity. The two are
different. Motivational imagination begins with questions like: What
would you do in this situation? If such-and-such happened to you, how
would you feel? These kinds of questions prompt us to imagine a real
situation, then analyze or rehearse our response.

THERE ARE FOUR LEVELS OF MOTIVATION.

To show how important imagination is in motivation, let's examine four
types of motivation and arrange them according to their power to affect
our actions. We'll go from weakest to strongest.

LEVEL 1:Compliance (doing what someone *makes* me do).
When my motive for doing something is to get an extrinsic reward or
avoid punishment, I am doing it from the motivation of compliance. It's
when my boss says, "If you want X, you will have to do Y." This could
be a threat or a bribe. It's based on the assumption that I wouldn't be
likely to do it unless spurred by external reinforcement. If I don't do
what is required, I will get written up or fired. If I do such and such, I
will get a prize or a bonus. Compliance is always in relationship to

some external authority who has the power to give or withhold rewards and punishments. In management it is often called the carrot-and-stick approach. This is level-1 motivation and represents the weakest motivation because a person will stay in compliance only as long as the authority is present and continues to give extrinsic rewards or punishments.

A workplace focused primarily on compliance is a paternalistic (adult-child) culture because managers are like parents who lay down the laws to children who had better obey them or else. Although compliance is a common feature of most work environments, we need to note that in terms of human motivation, it is the weakest, and places the responsibility for success on the shoulders of a controlling, paternalistic authority. Since the world is full of people who don't want to grow up and take responsibility, and plenty of others with an obsessive need to be in control, it often becomes the natural managing style.

LEVEL 2: Willpower (doing what I believe I *should* do).
The next level of motivation, synonymous with self-discipline, is when I do something on my own because I believe I should do it, even if I don't feel like it. Nobody is making me do it. I do it because I believe I should. It takes willpower to do something I believe I should, especially when I don't feel like doing it. Another word for willpower is self-discipline. I believe I should exercise in the morning. I set the alarm. When the alarm goes off, I am sleepy and it's cold outside. What I feel like doing is skipping it and staying in bed. But, like a drill sergeant, I tell myself: *Get up. Don't be a wimp. You promised yourself you would do this. You know you should. Come on, let's go!* When I do the thing I believe I should, all on my own, the reward is intrinsic. No one is there to congratulate me if I do or ridicule me if I don't. I pat myself on the back for my victory over my feelings. Psychologically, a life filled with such victories, whose rewards come from inside of me, builds my self-esteem and sense of competence, something compliance does not do.

Since we know that people are better motivated by values than compliance, a great deal of effort is being spent in companies to forge and communicate statements of core values intended to awaken the desire in employees to do the right thing whether authority is watching or not. Better that someone act from a sense of ethical imperative than fear or selfishness. The difficulty with this approach, however, is that values have to be internalized before they can become the source of self-discipline. They don't work hanging on the wall, especially in a culture of compliance. And employees are quick to become cynical if they do not see these values reflected in the behaviors of their leaders or in the actions taken by the company, especially in a crisis.

LEVEL 3: Imagination (doing what I *want* to because I *feel* like it). This is the most interesting, at least to me, because it is through imagination that my feelings are created in the first place. It is also through imagination that my feelings can be changed. We often hear it said that you should not make certain decisions on the basis of emotions. But that is very hard to do unless you are a master of self-discipline. If I can change my feelings, however, the required action will be much easier since I don't have to use sheer willpower to overcome them. When my feelings make me want to, instead of not want to, the motivation is much more powerful. That's why it occupies level 3 in the model. The startling truth is that imagination is more powerful than willpower.

Since this chapter is about the power of imagination to motivate, we will come back to this concept after looking at the final level of motivation.

LEVEL 4: Habit (doing what comes naturally)
Habit is the most powerful motivation of all, at level 4, because it is what we do without thinking. Obviously we don't do anything without thinking, in the technical sense. But when we use the phrase "I didn't think," we are speaking of force of habit. It's our knee-jerk response to stimulus. Habit is the result of all the programming we have absorbed in life and the repetitious responses to events. My force of habit is shutting the alarm off and going back to sleep when I said I would get up and exercise. My bad habits are all the things I do that seem to get in the way of my best efforts to achieve better health, increased knowledge, greater accomplishment, and more rewarding relationships. Our lifelong pursuit of competence and character is an effort to replace bad habits with good ones.

HABIT IS ANOTHER WORD FOR TALENT.

An interesting synonym for habit is talent. When we speak of ⌐
with a talent for working with handicapped children, we mean
someone who has developed certain attitudes and skills to such a
degree that the right responses emerge naturally and effortlessly. When
a response, good or bad, is automatic, it is a habit.

The most important job of a manager is getting the right people in
the right places doing the right things for the right reason. That's called
looking for and developing talent. Recruiting and keeping the best
talent is arguably the single most important skill for a manager. In order
to do this well, great managers do not leave the choice to the human
resources department. They know the most important skills needed in
every role and have learned that it is better to hire someone who already
has the talent (read habits), than to train someone who doesn't. Since
people love to do work that suits their talents, a good match means joy
in the workplace and virtually no supervision. Talent in a role means
the person can be trusted to solve problems, make decisions, and be
self-directed. The boss with a talented team can go play cards all day
and his department will probably outperform teams where motivation
is based on compliance and supervision. To reiterate a point made in
another chapter, great managers know they are not judged by what they
can do, but by what their teams can do without them. (Not that I
advocate managers leaving to play cards!)

For a delightful and energizing book that explores the relationship
between leadership, talent, and employee motivation, read *First, Break
All the Rules* by Buckingham and Coffman. An example of their
thinking:

> *Every* role, performed at excellence, requires talent, because
> *every* role, performed at excellence, requires certain *recurring*
> patterns of thought, feeling, or behavior. This means that great
> nurses have talent. So do great truck drivers and great teachers,
> great housekeepers and great flight attendants.[1]

"Recurring patterns of thought, feeling, or behavior" is the same as
habit. When something required is not easy for me, it's because I have

not developed the habit of doing it naturally. When I took my first tennis lessons, I was sure I would never be able to serve effectively. All the elements of the serve—the stance, the toss, the coordination of the tossing arm with the racquet, the shifting of the weight, the lifting with the legs, the bending of the back, the relaxation of the wrist, the contact point with the ball—felt unnatural to me. I was sure I could never learn to do it well. And for a long time I couldn't do it without thinking about each step. I looked awkward and felt clumsy. But the time eventually came when something that required so much concentration became as natural as walking. Now, when I serve, I just let it fly, comfortable in the knowledge that habit will take over, and it will be easy. What was once discouraging became fun because I got good at it and it had become habit.

Managers can't always be fortunate enough to find perfect matches of role and talent. So the second most important job of being a manager is developing and motivating people so they will have the habits that make for success in their role. How do you help people become motivated when they do not have the talent, or natural habits, for some important aspect of their job? The answer lies in the coaching talents of a manager. Not all managers have coaching skills as a talent. Many learn them on the job. Many others never learn them, stubborn in their habits of command and control that stem from feelings of insecurity. It is also these habits that keep such managers from hiring people with more talent than themselves for the role, or praising others as they develop their talents, or relinquishing decision-making authority to talented people.

IMAGINATION IS MORE POWERFUL THAN WILLPOWER.

Now that we have a clear understanding of the four levels of motivation, let's return to the subject of the chapter: imagination.

My wife, who was once the director of nurses for a rehabilitation hospital in California, asked one of her nurses one day to give a meditation at a staff meeting. The nurse brought a Shasta daisy and stood up in front of the room. She asked the members of the group to imagine that this flower represented their life and that each petal was something they were grateful for, something that made their lives

rewarding, meaningful, and fun. They were asked to w
thoughts on a piece of paper and share it with the person be
Then the nurse made a master list of "petals" on a flip chart. After doing
the exercise, the entire mood of the room was elevated. Counting one's
blessings is energizing and fun.

Then the nurse asked the question, "What will happen to these
beautiful petals, one by one, as you get old?" She went over to the flip
chart and pointed to the first item on the list. "What will happen to our
friends and loved ones?" she asked. "They will die." And she pulled out
some petals from the flower in her hand and let them flutter to the table
in front of her. "What will happen to our health? It will fail." More
petals fell.

She went through the list: job, home, car, recreation, shopping,
eating, reading, traveling, crafts, helping others, independence, etc. The
petals kept falling. Soon there was a profusion of disconnected petals
on the table. In the nurse's hand was a forlorn stem with a few lonely
petals remaining. The nurse then brought everybody's imagination to
the point. Holding up the pitiful remains of that beautiful flower she
said, "This is what is happening to our patients. Their lives were once
just like our lives: flowers in full bloom. They had all these lovely things
in their lives too. Think of the losses they have suffered. Think of all the
grief they have had to bear in giving up their petals one by one, some
all at once such as when they have a stroke. When my life looks like
this sad flower, I wonder what kind of person I will be. I hope I am
cheerful and cooperative and friendly to everyone around me. But I
have a feeling there will be days when I don't care about doing what my
nurses want me to do. There will probably be times when I will be
grumpy and depressed and angry. I may not respond the way others
wish I would. I might think they don't understand because, look at
them, they're all in the prime of life. Their flowers are full. They have
no idea."

Then the nurse looked over the group and said, "When I think of
this flower and my life, I *do* have an idea. Although I haven't walked in
their shoes, I can *imagine* what they are going through, and I feel so
fortunate to be an important part of their lives even when they're
difficult."

My wife shared this experience over dinner nearly 30 years ago, and it is still vivid in my mind. Our little family did the exercise together at the table. As we did, I thought about an old aunt I had stopped visiting in the nursing home because she was so crabby. That weekend, and many more, we went to see her, and I have never looked at an elderly person in the same way since.

That is the power of imagination to motivate. We can be threatened or bribed into treating people with respect: the motivation of compliance. We can have value statements on the wall that encourage us to be kind and loving even when we don't feel like it: the motivation of values and willpower. These motivations have their place and are useful, but this nurse demonstrated that neither is as powerful in motivating as imagination. Imagination influences feelings and feelings are the wellspring of desire. When we desire to do something from the depths of this well, it makes our actions easy and natural and real.

Compassion, caring, comforting, and kindness—which make up the bulk of adjectives linked to patient loyalty—are rooted in one's capacity for empathy. According to Webster's *New World Dictionary,* "empathy" is "the ability to share in another's emotions or feelings." It is composed of two Greek words that mean "affection" and "feeling." When people receive empathy, they feel loved and cared about. In other words they sense our compassion.

It is our ability to imagine what someone is going through that generates empathy. Acts of kindness, caring, and compassion, then, stem from imagination. Survivors of the Holocaust have done an exhaustive and systematic study of the "righteous gentiles" who risked their lives to save Jews in Germany and other countries during Nazi occupation. They found no correlation between taking this risk and one's religious beliefs. There was no correlation between it and conscientiousness, or morality. The only thing that correlated with the willingness to risk one's life for another was empathy. Living by values, moral beliefs, ethics, or religious teachings, according to the research, did not appear to predispose people to put themselves in jeopardy for another's suffering if they were outside their own families or congregations. The righteous few who dared to do these acts of courage for complete strangers came from every religion—and non-religion.

They spanned the entire range from self-sacrificing to self-indulgent people. Certainly Oskar Schindler of *Schindler's List* was no paragon of virtue or morality. The only common characteristic that could be found was a capacity for empathy that was strong enough to overcome the primitive fear for one's own safety.

On the opposite end of the religious spectrum from Schindler, one might think of Mother Teresa, a world-recognized symbol of compassion and empathy for the poorest of the poor. Certainly she was religious. Certainly she was a paragon of virtue. Did she not do her selfless acts of charity from a sense of moral imperative? According to her biographers, Mother Teresa's motivating force was based on a particular statement made by Jesus to His disciples in a lengthy passage about being kind to strangers who are sick, poor, hungry, imprisoned, or naked. He said, "Inasmuch as ye have done it to one of the least of these my brethren, ye have done it unto me." Mother Teresa says that this text was ever in her thoughts, and when she caressed and cradled the diseased form of a human being cast off by society to die in rags and filth, she imagined she was doing it to Jesus. She taught this same imagination to all her followers. She would say to them, "I see Christ in every person I touch because He has said, 'I was hungry, I was thirsty, I was naked, I was sick, I was suffering, I was homeless and you took me in.' It is as simple as that. Every time I give a piece of bread, I give it to Him. That is why we must find a hungry one, and a naked one." Imagination creates empathy, which leads to compassion. Values and ethical beliefs alone cannot do this because in them is not where human passion resides.

An emergency department nurse once said to me, "I don't like how our staff talks about some of the patients in our department. Behind their backs they make fun of the homeless and the uneducated and the drug addicts and people like that. I think how we talk about people affects how we treat them."

I asked her why she felt this way and the others didn't. She said, "I don't know. It's just that when I see one of these poor souls I think there but for the grace of God and two paychecks goes me."

This nurse finds empathy in certain situations where her coworkers do not. The difference, even though she didn't realize it, was imagination. Her thoughts (imagination) of what it would take for her to be in the same condition as these patients engendered empathy. The imagination in the minds of her coworkers, on the other hand, led them to feel judgmental, superior, scornful, and indifferent to the needs of the same patients. Since they didn't let their feelings show, they saw nothing wrong in their attitude.

Liz Jazwic likes to say that in the emergency department she once ran in Chicago, nurses thought they could cure teenage pregnancy by rolling their eyes! We can teach people to be polite and we can have zero tolerance for rudeness, but compassion doesn't come from pronouncements or policies. The subtle signals of facial expression and body language are almost impossible to fake. People know when others are judgmental and disapproving when they are pretending to be courteous. Our real thoughts are more powerful than we realize and more visible to others than we like to think.

INSPIRATION AND ACTING PRINCIPLES ARE THE MISSING INGREDIENTS.

Many service programs in hospitals have been copies of programs offered in other service industries, such as hotels, restaurants, and airlines. Training companies are heavily marketing their programs to the service sector, which also includes hospitals. Hospitals that have adopted these programs often report lackluster enthusiasm on the part of caregivers. I think when we examine their emphasis and content, we can readily see why.

Programs that are not hospital based do not have compassion as their cornerstone. Courtesy is the cornerstone in their programs. The jobs they represent are easy to script and standardize. They teach what to say and not to say in routine "moments of truth."

I don't mean to trivialize such encounters, but they do not represent the intimate kinds of moments between caregivers and patients. Teaching hotel employees how to point the way to the bathroom is a far cry from teaching them what to say when inserting a catheter. Learning how to carry bags, unlock the guest's door, and wait for a tip is nothing like having to help someone get undressed and into bed, and then put in an I.V. while they are moaning in pain. Learning how to say a pleasantry like "Have a nice day" is quite different from knowing what to say when a family is heartbroken and grieving, as is common in a hospital. When trainers come from outside the hospital industry, it's no wonder nurses often feel insulted with the shallow content and lack of real-life examples of what they face.

For hospitals not to teach the role of empathy, or inspire compassion, is a colossal omission, because empathy has the capacity to heal by its effect on stress, and compassion is the primary influence behind patient loyalty. At companies like Nordstrom, Marriott or Southwest Airlines, it is not compassion, but courtesy, that drives customer loyalty. But for our patients it is empathy, caring, and compassion.

Don't get me wrong. We need some training in courtesy. We need courtesy behaviors spelled out if they are going to be required. Some people need to be taught to look up and maintain eye contact when listening to someone. (How they got a frontline job with that problem amazes me.) But courtesy should not be the primary reason we want our employees to experience the training. The feelings I would want hospital employees to have when leaving a training program are those of inspired motivation for being part of a cause that is greater than they can find in any other occupation: healing the hearts, minds, and bodies of broken people. I would want them to come away stirred by stories of caregivers who have won the hearts of patients and their families. They need to be touched by hearing what loyal patients say. I would hope they would learn, in addition to films and skits demonstrating courtesy behaviors, from examples of compassion. For these things to happen, they need to be shown the power of imagination to create empathy. With understanding they still need practice in the art of expressing empathy by acknowledging people's feelings. They need hospital stories to inspire them and hospital examples to relate to.

Another popular topic taught in service-excellence classes is body language. But, as my acting coach used to point out, a person can't think one thing and make the body do something else and have it be believable. It is futile trying to learn body language as a substitute for real feelings. And if the appropriate feelings are present, the behaviors will also be there naturally.

What comes out nonverbally is a reflection of what is going on in the person's imagination. If a caregiver is exasperated, it shows. If she thinks the patient is stupid or contemptible, she can try to keep it from showing by faking her expression and demeanor, but it will probably still show. If her mind is on what is going on at home or what her coworker just said to her, that will be evidenced in the overtones of her communication with the patient. What caregivers probably do not need are more lessons in how to behave. They need *acting* lessons in how to imagine and feel so that their behaviors "come from a real place," as we learned in acting class. Teaching body language is like trying to teach people the mechanics of laughing without anything funny in their minds. The laugh won't be very believable. Besides, in the real world, when would a person ever think to practice body mechanics without feelings, as is often taught in courtesy behaviors? And if the feelings *are* there, why would a person need to be conscious of nonverbal mechanics?

WHY YOU CAN'T FAKE IT EVEN IF YOU TRY.

The reason lie detectors are so effective is that the body reacts to a person's imagination, thoughts and feelings, not to conscious attempts to fool the machine through willpower. Blushing, for instance, is a nonverbal response to imagination. Who can make themselves not blush or blush on cue without regard to what is going on in their minds? The galvanic skin response that causes a needle to create a polygraph is body language like blushing. Who can really fake it very well? Most human beings have pretty good built-in lie detectors. Instead of learning how to fake it, let's learn how to come from a real place by asking such questions as:

What would it take for me to act like that?
What if this were my mother (or my father or sister or brother)?
How would I feel if this happened to me (or my spouse or child)?

These are not questions about morality or ethics. They are not questions about what we *should* do. They are questions that can be answered only by imagination. And in that moment of imagination, we are in tune with the emotional content of our patient's experience. In that moment we will say the right thing. Our facial expression will convey the appropriate concern and kindness. Our body language will naturally reflect our empathetic thoughts.

Knowing the principle doesn't mean it is easy to do in real-life situations. It takes practice. One day I arrived at the public park for my tennis lesson. My instructor, Charlie, was called away because his wife was having a baby. I was excited for Charlie but a little disappointed that I didn't have a lesson. The receptionist saw my disappointment and said, "You know, there's a guy hitting the ball against the wall. He might like to play with you."

I went out and met the young person, a teenager. He seemed pleased about my offer and we warmed up on the court. Everything was going along fine until we decided to start playing for points. The first time he missed a ball or hit one out, he said, "Stupid!" to himself. I didn't think much of it at first, but as the set progressed, his self-recriminations became more vocal and angrier. After a while he was stomping his feet and shouting, "Stupid, stupid, stupid—you idiot."

As this went on, I became a bit unnerved and wished I had not gotten myself into this match. Although he never directed his anger at anyone but himself, I was beginning to get irritated and thought maybe I would go over to him, as I used to with my children, and say, "Look, if you can't play nice, I don't want to play with you." Somehow I knew that wasn't the right thing to say. Then he did something that looked so ridiculous that I could hardly contain my laughter. He threw the racquet up in the air and when he tried to catch it, it bounced out of his hand, hitting his head and falling on the court. I turned around, pretending to look for a ball so he couldn't see me laughing.

Then the acting lessons about imagination that I try to teach in my seminars came into my mind. When you're upset at or don't like another person's behavior, ask this question: *What would it take for me to act like that?*

I asked myself that question in my mind. It's important here to note that through imagination we can experience things that have never happened to us. Although I can't think of a time, even as a child, when I acted like this boy was acting with his tantrums, I *could* imagine how such behavior might have started. So I tried that. At first I thought maybe he was overly competitive by nature. But I was nobody. Nobody was watching our match. There was nothing at stake. Competition couldn't explain this behavior, it seemed to me.

My next line of thought went a little deeper. I imagined having a father for whom nothing I ever did was right—someone who called me "stupid" and "idiot" every time I made a mistake. I even imagined having an older brother who could do no wrong, who was captain of the football team and a star of the basketball team. I pictured trophies on the mantel. Friday nights flashed through my mind when the apple of my father's eye, my brother, performed to crowds of screaming fans.

The picture in my mind got to me. A rush of empathy replaced my exasperation. I no longer felt like scolding this boy. His antics no longer looked funny to me. I felt sorry for a kid whose self-esteem is so bad that it is less painful to call himself stupid than to hear it from somebody else whom he is sure is thinking it.

When your imagination puts you in a sympathetic place with another person, you don't have to worry about what to say. The right thing will automatically come out. I don't remember my exact words, but they went something like this: "Joe, you are too hard on yourself."

"I am? What do you mean?"

"Well, the way you scold yourself for missing a point. If I were that hard on myself, I wouldn't enjoy playing at all." Silence. "I think you play just fine, certainly as well as I do. And I would have more fun if I didn't worry about you getting down on yourself."

He appeared to be thinking, then said, "OK."

And that was that. No more yelling. No more racquet throwing. No more anger. It was as if all he needed was permission to get off his own back and have fun.

You might think, *There is no way to know what is going on with someone else, especially a complete stranger.* And that's true. There's a good chance this boy does not have a father, or a brother, for that matter. He might be mentally deficient. He might have an emotional disability. He might be on some kind of medication that makes a person extremely irritable. I will never know the truth. But that is not the point here. Truth is not the purpose of this exercise. Its only purpose is to open up my imagination to possibilities. And when I phrase the question, "*What would it take for me to....?*" I will imagine something that creates empathy because we are all prone to rationalize where we are concerned and forgive ourselves. Imagination is the source of our feelings. Empathy is an emotional response that is at the root of love and morality. It is worth cultivating in life, and if you are on the frontlines of a hospital, it is one of the greatest healing skills in the entire arsenal of medical practice.

Once more let me emphasize that what is OK for most companies in the service sector is not good enough for hospitals. Courtesy training is not enough where a deeper connection is needed with people who are suffering emotional and physical pain.

USE IMAGINATION AS A COACHING TOOL

Dr. Glenn Bigsby III, the medical director of a hospital residency program who heard me talk about this model of the four levels of motivation, said he wanted to incorporate it into his curriculum for residents. One of the important concerns of a physician, he told me, is patient compliance. Studies done on patient compliance with physicians' orders are discouraging. After being discharged from the hospital, a large percentage of patients never do or stop doing what they were told, in spite of their promises to comply.

What he saw in this model was that putting the emphasis on compliance (because your physician tells you to) was the weakest motivation, yet it's the most common approach that physicians use. Trying to urge the person to exercise more self-discipline (because you know you should do it) might be better, but it's still not the best. According to this model, the most effective approach, and least used, is to help the patient visualize how the regimen works on the body's systems and the positive consequences of sticking to it.

Physicians and nurses who understand the power of imagination could help patients imagine what will happen if they faithfully stick to a prescribed regimen. Maybe patients could write a vivid description— and promise to read it often—of how they will feel as they gain ground on their disease. They might be urged to picture doing something they cannot do now but will be able to do eventually if they stay the course.

When the spouse or entire family is part of the patient's problem, they might need to be present to participate in the imagination exercise so they will be a better support for the patient. The task is not how to get the patient and family to comply as much as how to create an imaginary picture so rich in detail that it will motivate the patient and family to want to do the hard work it will take, and refuel the source of energy to keep it up. Getting them to want to is the goal because it aligns feelings with actions, requiring less self-discipline than when they are not aligned.

Managers can have the same impact on employees as Dr. Bigsby suggests physicians can have on their patients. Using a person's imagination is a coaching technique that is fundamental in athletic coaching. Research on imagination has shown that athletes can improve their physical skills just by visualizing the motion over and over. In some studies the athletes who imagine doing a skill improve faster than those who actually practice it—and in less time! The theory postulates that this is because in imagination every shot is perfect.

But here we are not talking about physical skills. We want to emphasize the *motivational* power of imagination and its ability to transform our attitude.

Let's take a little service-related coaching situation. A manager decides to observe from a discreet corner how Connie, the receptionist in radiology, is doing on the job. Connie sits at a desk with a computer. Beside her, separating her space from the waiting area is a long, high counter. She was hired because she had a friendly personality and a gracious manner. She also has computer skills, so she is able to work on reports between greeting patients.

As our manager observes Connie, he makes some notes. Connie rarely looks up from her computer until she comes to a good stopping place. Patients often have to wait many seconds for her to acknowledge them. If they try to get her attention, she puts her hand up and says, "Just a minute." When she's finally ready, she looks up and says, "Yes?" She hands them a clipboard and returns to her work quickly before the patient turns away. The manager notices several other events that need addressing. She brushes away a person who is desperate to contact her husband. She blurts out, "You're here for the GI series?" loud enough to be heard in the waiting room, obviously embarrassing the patient. She is not helpful when someone wants to know more about the procedure. Several people indicate they are sick or in pain, but Connie doesn't pay any attention. One lady says she is nervous about the procedure because she's afraid it will hurt. She wants to know how long it will take. Connie responds with, "Once you get in there, it won't take that long." To one patient she says, "Just take a seat and try not to worry so much. It will be just fine." When someone asks when they'll be taken, Connie sounds a little defensive and says, "Look, I'm doing the best I can here. I don't know when they'll be ready for you."

This is obviously a coaching moment. Most managers will say that Connie has never been told the expectations and priorities in her job. She just needs to be told what to do and how to do it. They would take a compliance approach. They would probably call Connie in and give her a list of do's and don'ts: (1) look up and acknowledge patients with a smile and a friendly greeting as soon as they walk up to the counter; (2) stop what you are doing on the computer, stand up so you are at eye level, and give them your full attention; (3) offer to help them with anything they need as you hand them the clipboard; (4) when they ask how much longer it will be, offer to find out; (5) be careful not to violate the patient's confidentiality by saying personal things about the procedure out loud, etc.

These cover the routine moments that happen with just about everybody. A standard list of courtesy rules and behaviors for them might suffice for Connie. But how is she going to respond to all the spontaneous situations that come up? She does not appear to have developed a talent for saying the right thing because her mind is on other work and not tuned in to the needs of her customers. The manager still has a list of things he wants to address. If he says he saw her do or say such-and-such, she is likely to become defensive and not open to criticism.

Here is where an exercise in imagination would help him coach Connie without making her feel defensive. He might call her into his office and say, "Connie, is there an older person in your life whom you dearly love, admire, and respect?" Connie nods. "Tell me about this person," her boss continues.

nie's face lights up as she describes an aunt that was wonderful growing up. When she is through, her manager says, "She sounds like a wonderful person, Connie. Now imagine that you are working at your desk on the computer. In your peripheral vision a person walks up to the counter. You glance sideways and of all things it is your aunt! What would you do and say?"

Connie says, smiling, "I guess I would jump up and I'd be so happy to see her, I would give her a hug."

"You mean you wouldn't just look up and say, 'Just a minute'?"

"I suppose not."

"And if your aunt said she didn't feel well?"

"I'd probably help her sit down and fill out the form."

"If she seemed anxious to call somebody?"

"I'd let her use my phone."

"If she seemed scared about the procedure and had no idea what to expect?"

"I'd want to help her find out. You know I get questions like that all the time. Is there a way we could get something printed on each procedure I could hand the patient?"

"That's a good idea. I'll bring it up at our staff meeting and see if we can get that to help you help the patients."

The conversation could go on like this until the manager has covered everything. Then he might say, "I care more about what our patients experience than you getting your reports done. I wish you would imagine your aunt every time a person comes up to your counter and act exactly as you would with her—except the hug, maybe."

The manager has gotten Connie to say what's important rather than hearing it from her manager. This is not a small difference. There is no defensiveness when Connie is making the suggestions herself. The secret of great coaching is getting the other person to see the point and say it so the manager doesn't have to. Besides, by getting Connie to imagine a real situation in which she is at her best, he has motivated her without resorting to parent-child language or threats. In the future if he sees Connie slipping with someone, he can simply say, "Now Connie, is that how you would treat your aunt?" And she would get the point without being scolded.

IMAGINATION AND EMPATHY ALSO DIFFUSE ANGER.

The critical element in effective anger management is empathy. Any time we can imagine the situation from the other person's point of view, we lower our own defenses and, in the process, defuse their anger.

Over the years I have had a particular interest in this subject. I have seen many approaches to dealing with irate customers. Some are better than others. Almost all of them have a major flaw. They try to use left-brain techniques for a situation that is being played out in the right brain. By "left-brain" I mean things like lists, acronyms, and logic. But anger and the corresponding feeling it arouses, defensiveness, are emotional states. What works on emotions is imagination. And the purpose of imagination is to overcome defensiveness with empathy. So empathy is the most important skill to teach in dealing with an upset or irate person. One of Stephen Covey's seven habits of highly effective people is "Seek first to understand, then to be understood."[2] Every person who is in a position to have to deal with upset people needs to ponder and understand why this principle works so effectively.

At Disney, we were taught the acronym LAST: (1) listen, (2) apologize, (3) solve the problem, (4) thank them. There are many other acronyms taught by other programs that have these essential steps in them. One list I saw had 12 steps in handling an angry person! How could you ever remember all those?

There are two problems with this approach, even when the steps are fewer. First of all, an acronym is hard to recall in the heat of an angry exchange. (*What was that word again? HELP? CARE? SHARE? LAST? LIVE? FIRST? I can't remember. And I only learned it last week!*) The second problem is with the step "apologize." Most people believe that an apology is using a particular word, like I'm "sorry" or we "apologize." But what is effective in an apology is not the words but the empathy in the words. Unless the person apologizing is coming from a real place of empathy, the words "I'm sorry" are worthless for defusing anger. How many times have you heard someone say in a stern voice, "Well, I'm sorry, sir, but that's your problem." Is that an apology? It has the words "I'm sorry" in it, but somehow it doesn't feel like an apology. Empathy in *any* words is better than no empathy in the *right* words.

In dealing with anger, like any other emotion, it takes connecting with the person's feelings, not staying detached and in charge. Compassion is what is needed in these situations too. Imagination is the key to supporting one's words with genuine empathy. The real test of a person's talent in handling an angry customer is when the angry person calms down and says, "Thank you for listening to me. You have been very helpful (or compassionate, caring, kind, etc.)." Then when they tell others about the experience, they will say, "They were so nice to me when I got upset." That is the response talented handlers get all the time. If, on the other hand, the person gives one of these responses, the effort was a failure:

"Oh, just forget it."

"Who is your supervisor?"

"I'm not going to argue with you."

"I don't have to take this."

"Yeah, right!"

Every employee being taught to deal with an angry person should be able instantly to diagnose what went wrong if he or she hears one of these remarks. Any of these responses immediately tells me that what is missing in my manner and tone of voice was empathy. And the reason there is no empathy is because I chose to stay detached and in control, thereby not allowing myself to feel what the angry person feels. I might well have used the words "sorry" and "we apologize," but no empathy came through the words to let the other person know I care. There is no way to fake empathy. Learning to say "I understand how you must feel" will not do it. There is only one way for empathy to come through. It is when I use my imagination to come from a real place, the same place as the angry person. When a person feels empathized with, he or she *will* cool down. It is an automatic human reaction to feeling understood, unless one is on drugs or alcohol or has received such a grievous injury that nothing can console the person. But those are the extremes. The vast majority of cases can be defused with genuine empathy. Better than teaching people to say "I'm sorry that happened," we should teach phrases that cause us to put ourselves in their shoes like "I would hate that too," or "If that happened to me, I would be very upset."

In some seminars I have heard teachers say that the way to get an angry person to lower his or her voice is to lower yours—the idea being that he or she will mirror what you do. It sounds sensible, but it's not quite true. The teaching probably came from someone who filmed and then studied videotapes of what people do who have a talent for defusing anger. They carefully wrote down everything they heard and observed on the tape. Let's pretend we are watching one of these tapes of a nurse with this talent. We notice that she listens carefully and sympathetically. When she speaks, she speaks softly. Then we see that when the angry person responds, his voice has softened too. Wasn't that great: she lowered her voice and the angry person did too! This must be the key. But what *really* caused the angry person to lower his voice? I can tell you from experience that it was *not* the nurse lowering her voice. It is the fact that when you feel empathy for a person, your voice *automatically* softens. In contrast, when you feel defensive, your voice gets more and more strident, escalating into a shouting match.

For example, try lowering your voice and saying something sarcastic to an angry person like "You think you're the only person I have to take care of today?" Or lower your voice and say, "This is ridiculous." Or lower your voice and say, "I don't have time for this." Do you really think the angry person will lower his or her voice when you say something quietly with no empathy in it? Of course not. So discard the notion that you need merely to lower your voice. It's the wrong emphasis. Concentrate instead on imagining something that makes you feel empathy for the angry person. If you feel it, the words that come out will be right and so will your tone of voice. It will be the tone of voice—not the words—that says, "I understand. I am on your side. I would feel the same way. I care very much about this."

IMAGINATION AND EMPATHY ARE ALSO KEYS TO TEAMWORK.

At Disney all supervisors and managers are required to do frontline work several days a year. They sweep sidewalks, empty trash, serve hot dogs, sell merchandise, take tickets, and help guests onto rides. This puts them in touch with what it is like to deal with guests every day. It helps managers empathize with cast members and understand things from their perspective.

A friend of mine, Jim Londis, at that time vice president for community services at New England Memorial Hospital in Massachusetts, tells in a magazine article about participating in a similar program their administrator, Frank Perez, had implemented:

> In the hospital where I work, those not involved in clinical care are asked to "walk in a nurse's shoes" from time to time. It is a hands-on program in which administrators, trustees, and other nonclinical people work with nurses in the care of patients. On my most recent "walk," an elderly Alzheimer's patient ready to go home needed to be bathed.
>
> While working with the nurse, I realized that what these nurses did every day was sacred, that these sick bodies were—in their own way—dwelling places for God's Spirit. In that smelly hospital room I had what theologians call an "epiphany"—an overpowering sense of God's presence. . . . I received the blessing.[3]

Disney offers an increase in pay to frontline cast members who work in other departments as part of their career development. They want them to experience as many jobs as possible and find the right match for their talents. They also do it to foster teamwork and mutual understanding of each other's roles. A clerk who works the registration desk at the Wilderness Lodge told me that she had spent a month working in housekeeping as part of her work experience.

"It sure changes your perspective," she said. "I got to see how hard they worked. I got acquainted with everybody in the department. When we had guests waiting for a room, and it seemed to be taking a long time, I used to call them and say, 'Can't you guys hurry up and give me a room? I have people here who have been waiting for over an hour.' Now, when I call, I'm really empathetic. I say, 'Hi, Irene, this is Alice. How are things going? We have some guests here who have been waiting for a room. I know you guys are awfully busy and you're trying as hard as you can, but do you happen to have an estimate I might tell our guests?' "

Hospitals may have a more difficult time doing this because so many of the jobs take clinical specialists, but much more effort could be made to get everyone familiar with the people and working situations at the other end of phone requests for internal service. There is no reason that nurses can't be rotated through all the nursing units, including getting some extra training that goes with ICU and emergency.

The director of nurses who makes sure her nurse managers and assistant nurse managers have worked all over the hospital, including the job of being house supervisor, has gotten a priceless boost in nursing leadership, teamwork, and flexibility. One nurse from intensive care, who worked for several days in the emergency department, found that her attitude was changed about demanding calls from the emergency staff trying to get a room for their patient. "I never realized how frustrating it is when you have no control over your patient flow! In the ICU we have so much more control than they do. Now that I have worked there, I am much more sympathetic to them," she said.

Imagination, having a good mental picture of what it is like to work in another department, is an effective way to improve teamwork, smooth out the rough edges of communication, and create a shared vision of serving the patient together, regardless of where you work.

1. Marcus Buckingham and Curt Coffman, *First, Break All the Rules: What the World's Greatest Managers Do Differently* (New York: Simon & Schuster, 1999), p. 71.

2. Stephen R. Covey, *The Seven Habits of Highly Effective People: Restoring the Character Ethic* (New York: Simon & Schuster, 1989), p. 235.

3. James J. Londis, "Touching Is Believing," *Adventist Review*, April 1, 1993, p. 32.

CHAPTER

CREATE A CLIMATE OF DISSATISFACTION

After it opened in 1955, Disneyland brought financial stability to the Disney enterprise for the first time in its 30 years of existence. Walt Disney was 53 years old. "It all started when my daughters were very young, and I took them to amusement parks on Sunday," he told Bob Thomas, his official biographer. "I sat on a bench eating peanuts and looking all around me. I said to myself, dammit, why can't there be a better place to take your children . . . ? Well, it took me about fifteen years to develop the idea...Disneyland isn't designed just for children. . . . I want Disneyland to be a place where parents can bring their children—or come by themselves and still have a good time."[1]

Walt Disney did not invent the carnival or amusement park, but he did take the experience, analyze it, imagine how much better it could be, and then built the world a new benchmark in entertainment. Disneyland was born out of his dissatisfaction with these "dirty, phony places, run by tough-looking people." He took the negative stereotypes of carnivals and turned them inside out. Instead of dirt and trash everywhere, he would have immaculate gardens and walkways that looked like a private park. Instead of tough-looking employees, he would project an all-American look, young men and women groomed and dressed like ladies and gentlemen. Instead of contraptions propped up for the weekend on shaky platforms, he would have permanent structures so stable and solid that no parent would have a moment's worry about safety. Instead of nothing for parents and grandparents to enjoy, he would create shows and restaurants and park benches and nostalgic rides that tell a story. In short he would destroy every negative stereotype and reshape the image of carnivals and amusement parks forever.

In the world of animation, Walt Disney was also never satisfied, even when his films were superior to all his competitors. He was the first to figure out how to put synchronized sound to a cartoon in *Steamboat Willie*. His studio was the first to use Technicolor in animation, and when the color chipped off, he and his staff worked long and hard to improve the composition of the coloring agent so it would adhere. When he went heavily in debt, yet again, to produce the first feature-length animation, *Snow White*, everyone was sure it would be a commercial flop. Cartoons were supposed to be less than 10 minutes long. According to conventional wisdom, nobody would sit through a feature-length animated film. But it won an Academy Award and was followed by many more features, which are still a staple of the American film industry. He and his brilliant creative staff invented the gadgets and techniques that combined live-action with cartoon characters in *Mary Poppins*.

The list of technological and creative inventions and "firsts" attributed to him and his "imagineers" fill the books on his life and accomplishments. After virtually every innovative commercial success, his competitors hired away his most creative and productive talent. Walt Disney constantly had to rehire, retrain, and continue with less experienced technicians and artists. He sold everything he had and faced bankruptcy many times to fund his next dream. Every accomplishment brought joy to his heart, but never complacency. He was never satisfied and was giving instructions for how to improve the plans for the Magic Kingdom and EPCOT Center in Florida, right up until his death from lung cancer in 1966. His brother, Roy, who saw the projects through to completion in 1971, never worked so hard in his life, and it was to complete another man's vision. He named the entire

complex Walt Disney World instead of Disney World
brother all the credit. He once looked to the heavens
exasperation, "Walt, what have you gotten me into?"

DISSATISFACTION IS THE FATHER OF IMPROVEMENT.

If necessity is the mother of invention, dissatisfaction must be the father
of improvement. Necessity may invent the mousetrap, but
dissatisfaction builds a better one. The curious truth is that being good
is the enemy of being great. Complacency is the adversary of excellence.

Martin Stankard, a national Malcolm Baldrige Award examiner who
trains other examiners, shares this formula for a culture of continuous
improvement and excellence:

$$\underset{\text{with "as is"}}{\text{Dissatisfaction}} + \underset{\text{"could be"}}{\text{Dream of}} + \underset{\text{of "how to"}}{\text{Knowledge}} > \underset{\text{INERTIA}}{\text{ORGANIZATIONAL}}$$

Dissatisfaction with the status quo, plus the dream of what
greatness would look like and the knowledge of how to get there, must
be greater than an organization's natural inertia. Notice that the formula
begins with dissatisfaction. How do you overcome the comfort zone of
personal and organizational inertia without being dissatisfied with the
way things are? Plus, all this has to happen *before* the hard work of
improvement can even begin.

Behavioral science confirms this equation. If I want to lose 15
pounds, it starts with dissatisfaction over my current state of being. In
addition, I will need to have a vivid picture of how I want to appear,
how my slacks will fit, how a flatter tummy will look, how much
younger people may think I am. Dreams give us the fuel for desire, the
energy to get up and do the work. Knowledge of how to lose 15 pounds
and keep it off permanently is also important. But my worst enemy is
going to be the kind of thinking that says, "Fifteen pounds doesn't really
seem *that* bad. I am actually in pretty good shape for a guy my age. We
all gain some weight when we get older. It's natural." Complacency is
the human equivalent of inertia.

At every level in an organization where there is work to do, this
formula for change applies—at the level of individual effort, at the unit

., at the division level, and even the highest level of administration. That's why it is important to cultivate an entire culture of dissatisfaction in order to maintain a momentum for improvement that leads to sustained excellence. Having a few stars who do it is not enough. A department here and there dedicated to improvement won't be able to lift the whole organization.

BEWARE OF A "POP PSYCHOLOGY" APPROACH TO CHANGE LEADERSHIP.

We are a culture that believes there must be an easier way to do anything. We come up to a challenge and want an easy way around it instead of the hard way through it. We are wooed by books and programs that promise quick and effortless solutions to something difficult. With such-and-such a supplement you can lose those pounds without exercising and still eat all you want. You can raise your self-esteem by writing affirmations and telling yourself in the mirror that you're wonderful. You can build muscle strength and tone with our electrical stimulator. You can build up your cardiovascular system in 10 minutes a day on our machine without breaking a sweat. You can simply "think" and grow rich, "think" and grow thin, "think" and get smart, "think" and play tennis, "think" and feel great about yourself.

The dream (the "think" part of these self-help approaches) is vital for improvement. We rarely accomplish anything without a dream, or great things without a vivid obsession. But there are many with the dreams who do not overcome inertia to follow through with the hard work. The dream alone takes you nowhere. If you want the muscles, you have to do the exercises.

The equivalent in leadership psychology is the notion that creating a dream of greatness is the vital ingredient that is missing in most organizations. First, hospitals went through exercises in writing mission statements. When that did not move organizational inertia, we decided we needed statements of core values. Then it was vision statements. We weren't making our mission statements and core values vivid enough. Lance Secretan says our problem is that all these vision statements lack inspiration. He says inspirational leadership is what is needed and that people do not work for a mission, they work for a cause. Semantics aside, it takes the whole formula to overcome inertia.

Vision alone, regardless of what we call it, is not enough to muster the huge effort it takes to defeat the inertia of standard practices, bureaucratic structures, systems, and management processes. We still need a relentless dissatisfaction with our performance and a map of how to improve, to get up finally and scale the walls, move the mountains, dam the rivers, and drain the swamps that stand in the way of true greatness. It has to be relentless because being the best, or being the greatest, is not done in a day or a month or a year. Ask any accomplished athlete. He might tell you about the dream he has had since childhood, but the truth is, the hard work of reaching that dream is relentless. And even if he breaks a world record, he is still not satisfied! Never being satisfied is the driving force behind individual effort. And, we might add, corporate effort.

THE ROLE OF STATISTICS AND SCOREKEEPING SHOULD BE TO CREATE DISSATISFACTION.

The foundation for creating a climate of dissatisfaction is the desire and willingness to know the unvarnished truth about performance. The only way to have an accurate picture of performance is to keep some kind of score by applying numbers to each aspect of performance that must be executed to reach a goal. A world-class tennis player is interested in more than the final score of his tennis matches. He (or at least his coach) is interested in the numbers that describe various parts of his game. What percentage of first serves went in? What percentage of points did he win when he went to net? When he stayed back? When he hit a forehand? A backhand? What was the ratio between aces and double faults? Between winners and unforced errors?

Winning is the goal, but analysis of the game provides the information for improvement. All winning and no losing would breed complacency. A great player is not interested in a coach who tells him only how good he is. He is more interested in one who tells the truth about his performance and what it will take to improve. In doing so, the coach capitalizes on the athlete's dissatisfaction coupled with his dream of greatness. Of course, along the way, there are constant pats on the back to keep the fires burning.

Likewise, without keeping score and putting numbers to aspects of departmental performance, a manager loses his best source of motivation for constant improvement. As was pointed out in chapters 2 and 3, at Disney every facility and resort keeps track of constantly updated scores on guest perceptions. Overall perceptions are not good enough. Guest perceptions on every aspect of their visit are measured and posted backstage in large print for all cast members to see every day. When I wondered why Disney doesn't combine the fours and fives in measuring overall satisfaction, the person I asked said something quite telling: "They would all be 99 or 100 percent, and what would that tell our cast members? They are perfect!" In other words, Disney doesn't want cast members resting on their laurels as a world-class organization with nothing to improve. Dissatisfaction is much more motivating than complacency.

REACHING THE 100TH PERCENTILE DOES NOT MEAN WE HAVE ARRIVED.

When I go to healthcare conferences on patient satisfaction, the star performers talk in terms of being in a certain percentile in patient-satisfaction scores. This means that compared to other hospitals in the same database, their scores are in a certain percentile. "We were at the 14th percentile on the Press Ganey and set a goal to be at the 85th percentile by the end of last year," they will say. "This year our goal is to reach the 99th percentile."

All progress should be applauded. But what happens when they reach a goal like the 99th percentile? They will be able to tout their scores nationally. They will be able to create the impression that patients will be completely satisfied when they are admitted to their hospital. Most employees view 100 percent as perfection. They are likely to believe they have reached the ultimate goal. Any more pushing to improve might be seen as senseless when you are already at the top.

However, let's take a look at what it really means in terms of patient satisfaction and loyalty to be at the 99th percentile. According to the Healthcare Advisory Board's research, the 99th percentile for hospitals would mean that only about 60 percent of patients are "very satisfied" with their care!

The Disney organization does not try to motivate employees by trying to make them look better than they are. They are not in a national guest satisfaction database with other resorts and theme parks. They do not use comparative percentiles with their employees to prove they are better than Sea World or Universal Studios. They simply put out the stark facts about what percentage of guests are "very satisfied" with their care on a scale of one to five. It is the unvarnished truth that creates a culture where "good isn't good enough" and "we can always do better."

Competition is not a better motivator than our own deepest desire to be more competent tomorrow than we are today. In his book *Understanding Psychotherapy* Michael Franz Basch cites considerable research on infant development before concluding:

> My emphasis here on the search for competence as fundamental for behavior marks a definite departure from a concept that underlies much of the literature in dynamic psychiatry: namely, Freud's theory that all behavior has as its goal the pleasure that attaches to the discharge of . . . energy generated by a sexual or an aggressive instinct. That there is a more scientific explanation than the instinct theory, which Freud himself called the mythology of psychoanalysis, . . . is buttressed by these experiments which demonstrate that even in infancy the search for competence is the prime motivator for behavior, and that its attainment is the basic source of pleasure.[2]

In other words, the drive for competence is the primary source of pleasure in the normal development of a human being. When it is constantly thwarted, given up, or displaced, psychiatric intervention is often needed.

There is pleasure attached to competence. Often competition can stimulate people to excel, but it is a distortion of our basic drive if winning is more important than the pleasure of achieving higher levels of competence. In the right atmosphere of teamwork, coaching, and learning, constant improvement is fun—just as improving one's athletic skills can be more exhilarating than actual competition.

ADOPT THE MOTIVATIONAL CYCLE OF CONTINUOUS IMPROVEMENT.

W. Edwards Deming introduced some graphical tools of statistical analysis to the relatively uneducated workers of industrial organizations. It worked such wonders in Japanese companies that he is acknowledged throughout the world as the father of the quality revolution. It may have seemed like a revolution to Japan's competitors in America, but it took about six years of sustained effort before it "suddenly" became as visible as a tidal wave to the rest of the world.

Deming understood the refueling effect that measurement, dissatisfaction, and improvement have on human motivation. Most of the statistical tools Deming taught were adopted from the writings of Walter Shewhart, a quality analyst at AT&T in the 1930's. Deming's great contribution was not so much in original statistical approaches, but in his keen understanding of human motivation and the barriers to improvement that exist because of poor management systems and the American penchant for command and control structures that seemed to work so well in the crisis of World War II.

One of Shewhart's models became a cornerstone of Deming's teachings. It was the cycle for continuous improvement, often referred to as the PDCA (Plan, Do, Check, Act) cycle. There are many variations in the words used, but the cycle is a fundamental concept in performance improvement. Basically it pictures a heavy sphere moving up an incline by rotating constantly through the steps of planning, implementing, measuring, being dissatisfied with the results, and starting the cycle over again. Over time, the results keep improving and the ball progresses up the incline toward perfection, which is always just out of reach. The point here is that it takes *being dissatisfied with current results* to keep the ball from resting in a state of inertia or rolling backward. What inspires and motivates and is ultimately gratifying to people is the *positive trend* they see over time, which makes all their cyclical efforts worthwhile.

A good example is the effort made by the radiology department of Florida Hospital East Orlando. The director, Lester Rilea, ran a busy department, with just four rooms, that was doing 42,000 radiology procedures a year for the entire hospital, including emergency and outpatient. They worked as quickly as they could but did not know exactly what their average turnaround time was. They started with emergency procedures (completed procedure minus the time the procedure was ordered) which represented about 25,000 procedures. More than 50,000 patients pass through the emergency department (ED). The average radiology turnaround time was 40 minutes. The national benchmark, according to the Healthcare Advisory Board, was 25 minutes. The department had every right to be satisfied with their comparison since they did not have digital equipment and had such a heavy load on just four rooms, none of which were attached or dedicated to the ED.

But Rilea was not satisfied. Neither was his staff. They wanted to see what they could do to improve their performance without adding staff, space, or new equipment. The first thing they did was to post measurement results where everybody could see them, and ED turnaround time was added to everyone's performance expectations from director to technical staff.

Then they reorganized the workload so that there was more teamwork in transporting patients, hanging films, and answering the phones.

Performance was also graphed by time of day to identify times when bottlenecks frequently occurred. By adjusting staffing for these load times, productivity improved about 7 percent, measuring examinations per hour worked.

A board was put up with slots to track manually where each procedure was in the schedule and how many were waiting to be done. This allowed the supervisor to allocate staff time more efficiently.

Any procedure taking more than 30 minutes was analyzed for reasons why and ways to decrease the time. This resulted in more noticeable improvements.

Finally they further shortened the time by having all radiographs placed on a multiviewer in the ED where emergency physicians could look at them before the radiologist provided a final reading.

These and other efforts helped the department match the national benchmark in less than a year. This meant a 38-percent reduction, which translated into a time savings of 5,000 hours per year to the ED and its patients. Think of the double win this effort garnered for the hospital: happier ED patients (they received the highest satisfaction scores of any step reported on ED surveys) and a sizeable savings in the bottom line. The last I heard they are even surpassing that.

What is important about this example is that the pressure to reduce radiology turnaround time for emergency patients was not driven by edicts from top management. It was driven by a staff that was dissatisfied with average performance and wanted to be the best in the nation—this in spite of serious space limitations, high patient volume, old equipment, and staffing constraints.

The literature is filled with stories like Rilea's from all departments in healthcare. Any department manager interested in what others are doing can readily get benchmarking information and process-improvement ideas. Many present their improvement stories at national conferences. The most successful efforts, like those of Rilea and his staff, are self-imposed and continuous. They represent departmental cultures in which dissatisfaction with the status quo generates excitement and excellence.

To prepare for his highly acclaimed, best-selling book, *Good to Great,* Jim Collins and a team of researchers spent 10 man-years of careful analysis to find out how some long-standing companies made a monumental leap at a critical juncture in their history that left their competitors in the dust. He called this event "going from good to great." The most startling finding of the research was that what looked like a leap to competitors and investors was simply the visible breakout of an almost imperceptible effort of relentless improvement related to the core competencies of their business. He labeled this phenomenon the "flywheel effect."

> No matter how dramatic the end result, the good-to-great transformations never happened in one fell swoop. There was no single defining action, no grand program, no one killer innovation, no solitary lucky break, no miracle moment. Rather, the process resembled relentlessly pushing a giant

heavy flywheel in one direction, turn upon turn, building momentum until a point of breakthrough, and beyond.[3]

Applying lessons gleaned from the inspirational account of Admiral Jim Stockdale's eight-year ordeal as a prisoner of war in Vietnam, Collins also found in the good-to-great companies something he named the "Stockdale Paradox."

> Every good-to-great company embraced what we came to call the Stockdale Paradox: You must maintain unwavering faith that you can and will prevail in the end, regardless of the difficulties, AND *at the same time* have the discipline to confront the most brutal facts of your current reality, whatever they might be.[4]

Dissatisfaction with the brutal facts about one's current reality, then, is a prerequisite to breakthrough performance, which precedes greatness.

WHAT ABOUT EMPLOYEE SATISFACTION?

In being immersed in the Disney culture, I did not notice a strong focus on employee satisfaction. There was not an unusual expenditure of effort to make employees happy. Employee-satisfaction surveys were conducted. Some managers chose to do 360 evaluations on themselves for self-discovery and personal improvement. But I did not get the impression that Disney existed to satisfy employees. Employees existed to satisfy Disney guests. Wages were thought by most employees to be low compared to other places. There was no tolerance for employees who deviated, even slightly, from cultural norms. Behavioral standards were exacting and strictly enforced. Youthful exuberance was a desirable quality, but not if it bordered on defying authority or making fun of the culture. Even peer pressure was directed at toeing the company line.

The first bits of company gossip I heard from fellow employees had to do with what you had better not do if you want to stay employed. One swear word, for instance, spoken on stage, even if no guest hears it, is grounds for immediate firing. Walt Disney once fired a colleague on the spot for using a four-letter word that only Walt heard. So the stories went.

I heard about the guy who took a friend backstage into the tunnels and was fired for that. Another took pictures backstage—and was gone. Whether any of these stories are true or not, I'll never know, but they are the kinds of stories cast members tell that let you know you'd better love working here and follow the rules. Even the union, it was said, will not come to your rescue if you are dismissed for violating a customer-service standard. For things like rudeness or profanity, there was no three-strikes-and-you're-out policy.

Over the course of two careers that spanned 30 years, I do not remember ever being reprimanded. Yet, within my first six months at Disney I was reprimanded three times. The first time happened on my first day. I walked up to the registration desk for Disney Traditions, the two-day orientation to Disney's expectations and service standards. The person at the desk looked up and asked, "Where is your coat?"

"In the car," I replied. It was a scorching, hot, humid day.

"You'll need it to enter class," she said. "And if you are not back by eight o'clock we will have to reschedule you for another time, because facilitators close the doors right at eight."

I dashed to my car. I remembered the sheet of paper I had received that clearly spelled out the attire I was supposed to wear for orientation. It specified for men: a jacket with lapels, shirt with a collar, dress slacks with leather belt, and leather shoes (no tennis shoes), with socks. I had wondered when I read it how they thought they could get teenagers, who would be working in an amusement park all day in the hot sun, serving guests dressed in shorts and tee shirts, to dress like that for orientation! As I returned to the casting center where my class was to be held, I saw several young people headed back to their cars, turned away at the door for improper dress.

The second reprimand came a couple of months later when my boss, Steve Heise, told me that I would have to cut my hair because a little wisp of it tended to curl out over the top of my ear.

The third time came from a fellow cast member, a peer, who said she had seen me in the park walk right over a piece of paper. "You are at Disney, now," she said. "You need to act like it and set a good example."

This certainly did not sound like a place that coddles its employees and cringes in fear that someone might get their feathers ruffled and threaten to leave.

Disney expends a great deal of money and effort to recruit and keep the right people. But their attraction is not pay or benefits or special goodies for cast members. It is in finding self-motivated people with enthusiasm for creative opportunities and an unabashed love for putting a smile on other people's faces. In the words of Jim Collins, they, like all truly great companies, work hard to "get the right people on the bus," but are equally vigilant in working hard to get "the wrong people off the bus." The ones who stay have a fanatical devotion to creating a magical experience for children and adults of all ages and from all cultures. The ones who leave are the detractors, the cynics, the indifferent. For them, Disney is not a great place to work. They are not comfortable in a culture in which even their peers will call them on a cultural infraction. If you talked to any of them, you would not think Disney placed a high value on employee satisfaction.

It appears we have a paradox. We desire satisfied employees, but we also want employees who are never satisfied with the status quo and will lift the organization to new heights of greatness. Maybe satisfaction is something like happiness. If you make it your primary goal, it escapes you. But if you seek things like knowledge, goodness, service, integrity, and self-mastery, it may result in deep satisfaction.

DOES EMPLOYEE SATISFACTION PRECEDE PATIENT SATISFACTION?

Though studies have shown that there is a strong correlation between employee satisfaction scores and patient satisfaction scores, it does not necessarily mean that improving employee satisfaction will improve patient satisfaction. It could just as easily be true that in focusing on the patient's experience and uniting in a successful effort to improve patient satisfaction and loyalty, we will reap the bonus of raising employee satisfaction.

In Ray E. Brown's 1966 classic *Judgment in Administration*, arguably the most insightful book on hospital leadership ever written, he addresses this notion:

> The great concern demonstrated over employee happiness and satisfaction may be based to a large extent on a misapprehension. We are prone to think that if something has a strong negative influence, its opposite will have an equally strong positive influence. Thus, we have a tendency to think that if unhappy and dissatisfied employees are poor workers, then happy and satisfied employees should be good workers. This proposition suffers on two counts. In the first place, it assumes an all-or-none quality for happiness and satisfaction. People are not limited only to happiness or unhappiness, satisfaction or dissatisfaction, about things. They can also be indifferent. The area of indifference is perhaps a much larger one than the total of the two extremes. In most matters it probably makes little difference whether the individual is happy so long as he is not very unhappy. In the second place, the assumption relies on a non-sequitur. Because I may not work hard if I am dissatisfied, it does not follow that I will work hard if I am satisfied. I may simply dislike hard work. Whatever connection there is between good performance and satisfaction, it is likely that satisfaction is the dependent variable and is the result, rather than the cause, of good performance. An individual who gets away with shoddy performance is likely to become an unhappy and dissatisfied individual.

None of this is intended as an argument against the responsibility of administration to provide as much satisfaction for every job as is consistent with acceptable performance by the individual and with the resources of the enterprise. It merely argues that being satisfied is not the final determinant of satisfactory performance.

A legitimate concern of a great service organization is that trying to please employees can sometimes run counter to pleasing your customers. Which comes first? Disney would subscribe to the theory, although I did not see it written anywhere or spoken of, that customers come first and employees come second when you are considering any action that affects either one.

Let me give an example. Hospitals often set up committees to make suggestions for improving employee morale. Many times their recommendations include relaxing dress codes. They may reason that the dress code is too conservative. That people should be free within reason to dress as they please. That clothes do not make the person and regimentation is stifling. That there is no consistency in the current policy anyway. That managers don't like to enforce dress codes and employees resent it if they do. So the logic goes, and it's easy to be persuaded.

At Disney, the "appearance guidelines" (strictly enforced!) are determined by customer expectations, not employee satisfaction. Employees who take pride in the Disney organization's obsessive dedication to making the best possible impression on guests, understand this, and would never whine about their lack of freedom to express themselves. The right people on the Disney bus would not chafe under a dress code clearly based on guest expectations. If you're a cynic, you might hate it, but cynics should get off the Disney bus. They certainly shouldn't be allowed to take over the bus.

A compromise motion also seems to come out of these committees with some regularity. In most places it's called "casual Fridays," and is common in many companies. If we don't want to loosen our daily dress code, why don't we at least give people their freedom of expression one day a week. Is that too much to ask? We have read in the media how effective this seems to be for boosting morale in other workplaces. Why wouldn't it do the same for us?

Guess what Disney would say to such a request? The same thing hospitals need to say: "Guests who come on Friday are just as important as those who come on Monday. For them it could well be their only contact with our company. What makes the impressions of one-seventh of our customers less important than the rest?" The right people on the bus would agree. They would be just as jealous for the reputation of their company on Friday as any other day.

Of course even the most dedicated people can be persuaded to adopt a misguided idea. When you consider where the idea comes from, it is easier to understand why many get drawn to something that seems so harmless. The technological revolution of the last two decades has been stunning. Those of us in the service sector have watched with envy as employees in hundreds of Silicon Valley start-ups and dot-com ventures became rich overnight. Talent from all over the world flocked to these companies, where they reported being so energized that they worked day and night for the success of their venture. Morale in these places soared, and so did creativity and drive. Everyone wanted to be part of something exciting. The media wrote endearingly about the free-wheeling cultures that allowed people to think and act outside the box. We read about how liberating it was for employees to come to work in frayed shorts and a tee shirt if they wished. How nobody ever wore a tie and you could wear nose rings or sport tattoos or let your hair grow as long as you liked. We were given to believe that this helped free the human spirit that was so stifled in the up-tight cultures of traditional corporate America.

Any hospital employee, or Disney cast member for that matter, could easily be persuaded that freedom from dress restrictions would have a positive impact on morale. After all look what it is doing in these exciting places. But in all the praise about these unfettered cultures, we can easily lose sight of the single biggest difference between their customers and ours: *Their customers never actually see their employees.* How people look to each other in a workplace where customers do not see them doesn't matter much. If an insurance company wants to have casual Fridays or abolish the dress code, who cares? Their customers are on the phone, not sitting or lying in front of them. If a web-based catalog service has scruffy-looking employees, what does it matter? They do not see each other face to face. Customers do not walk down the halls of companies where employees are writing software. They do not rub shoulders with service-center personnel when they are online about a computer problem.

But that is not the way it is with our patients in the hospital, or Disney's guests in its resorts and theme parks, or Marriott's patrons in its hotels and restaurants. Here, the customer comes face to face with the employees who represent the company, and their first impressions are often their most lasting impressions.

I will never forget the shudder I felt when a hospital CEO in Colorado told me why he felt compelled to take away casual Friday after he had approved it. One Halloween a family had asked to see him in his office. Their daughter had died in the operating room, and the person who gave them the tragic news was a nurse dressed up like a clown. The incongruity of the moment was deeply disturbing to the family. And the CEO never wanted to take the chance that such an encounter could happen again.

The determining question regarding all suggestions in a service industry should be "How will this affect the perceptions of our customers or guests?" Their impressions always come first and are an important key to their continued loyalty.

Don't get me wrong. I care deeply about creating an environment in which employees love to work. Poor managers who cannot relate with integrity and caring to their employees, who create needless bureaucracy to bolster their needs for superiority and control, need to be taken off the bus too. Every effort should be made to find and promote managers who know how to recruit and keep the right people, who create high morale through a shared dream of superior service carried out by a team of people with a passion for excellence. Finally, we need managers who can create a culture in which workers are so motivated that they are rarely satisfied with the status quo and find pleasure in continuous improvement.

---

1. Bob Thomas, Walt Disney: *An American Original* (New York: Simon & Schuster, 1994), p. 11.

2. Michael Franz Basch, *Understanding Psychotherapy: The Science Behind the Art* (New York: HarperCollins Publishers, 1988), p. 27.

3. Jim Collins, *Good to Great* (New York: HarperCollins Publishers, 2001), p. 14.

4. Ibid., p. 13.

5. Ray E. Brown, *Judgment in Administration* (Chicago: Pluribus Press, 1982), p. 73.

CHAPTER

CEASE USING COMPETITIVE MONETARY REWARDS TO MOTIVATE PEOPLE

Many years ago, on a plane from Kansas City to Los Angles, I was impressed by the outstanding personality and graciousness of a flight attendant. When I got a chance, I said to her, "You're terrific. I was impressed by the way you handled that woman who was so upset."

The flight attendant thanked me and a few minutes later came back with a little compliment card with her name carefully filled in on one of the blanks. "That was such a nice thing you said about me," she said. "Would you mind putting your remarks on this card? If I get enough cards, I might win a vacation to Hawaii."

I filled out the card, but as I did so, something didn't feel right. The kindness I had witnessed seemed tarnished. As I looked at the card, I began to doubt the sincerity of her actions. I didn't like the cynical thoughts this card aroused, but I couldn't help it. In analyzing what had just happened from a psychological point of view, I envisioned a possible chain reaction of unintended consequences that could easily outweigh any gains (if indeed there were any gains worth getting) from an individual competitive-reward system designed to improve customer service.

1. Somebody in management knows you can get more of a desired behavior if you offer a reward or monetary incentive.

2. Somebody in management also believes that people will outdo themselves and go the extra mile if you make rewards competitive.

3. Employees who are truly talented at reading and handling the emotional reactions of their customers and teammates will automatically know that participating in the reward system will breed cynicism and rivalry between team members and might even render suspect the moment of kindness in the customer's eyes. Consequently the best relators will probably not hand out the cards.

4. In the end the people who turn in the cards and win the reward will be resented, not admired. This will diminish the spirit of great teamwork in which they respect each other and pitch in to help each other succeed.

5. The manager will not likely see the unintended negative consequences because he or she will notice only the many cards that were turned in, thus validating the "effectiveness" of the reward system.

6. The winners may actually be the least sensitive people on the team, but their cards will earn them special praise and recognition.

7. The insensitive person who has won the prize and alienated her coworkers is now seen as outperforming her peers and will eventually be promoted into management.

8. Since it worked for her, and since her competitiveness was rewarded, she will manage in the same way, and the cycle of trying to motivate people with competitive rewards will be perpetuated, as it is in many organizations.

Any manager considering a reward system designed to motivate people to give better service needs to examine these eight potential outcomes and consider the long-range consequences of shifting the employee's focus from intrinsic values to extrinsic rewards—and from cooperation to competition. This is not a minor shift. It is a shift that has dramatic consequences, mostly negative, on corporate cultures. It underscores the authority of those who dispense the rewards and tell people what to do, reinforcing a culture of compliance and hierarchy. It is certainly not compatible with transformational leadership or servant leadership models that are proving their value in today's companies.

COMPETITION AND REWARDS
ARE WIN/LOSE THINKING.

Business practices are often years behind business thinking. Organizational inertia and long-standing practices are hard to break, even when everybody believes the old system is not very effective. Stephen Covey's book, *Seven Habits of Highly Effective People*, has been a best seller since 1990. In fact it has been reported that no nonfiction book has ever sold so many copies in so short a time as this book. Added to the hundreds of companies that have participated in Covey's leadership seminars, listened to his tapes, and underlined his manuals, you would think individual competitive rewards like pay for performance, merit pay, employee of the month, and a host of other practices would be virtually gone by now. In *Seven Habits* he chastises managers who are "trying to get the fruits of cooperation from a paradigm of competition."[1]

Covey's model has three human developmental stages: (1) dependence, (2) independence, and (3) interdependence. Stage three is the most mature stage and represents the real world after our education. Schoolchildren and young adults compete for grades and establish their independence by showing what they have learned independently. But as soon as an adult enters the mature world of marriage, family, and work, he enters an interdependent reality. The competitive activities whereby people learn and establish their individual competencies and independence no longer work as they used to and are actually a hindrance to success in an interdependent reality. As Covey says, "The moment you step from independence to interdependence in any capacity, you step into a leadership role."[2]

Leaders are people who work with others to create a win-win environment at home and at work. However, according to Covey and other experts on corporate culture, "The spirit of Win/Win cannot survive in an environment of competition and contests."[3]

It is generally believed that salespeople are a unique breed: highly competitive and driven by the desire to be number one and beat out their peers for a trip to Bermuda or some other grand prize. According to conventional wisdom, sales organizations have to use contests to motivate and get the maximum production from its sales force. Covey cites several examples that dramatically disprove that notion, in which sales companies have far exceeded all their previous sales records when rewards were based on teamwork instead of individual competition and most salespeople felt like winners instead of only a few.

I choose to reference Covey instead of other significant writers on the subject because even managers and administrators who do very little reading on the topic of leadership have read his famous book. His influence has been enormous, yet the rewards systems he has strived to eradicate so organizations can move from rivalry to synergy are still the norm in most companies and certainly in most hospitals. And committees assigned the task of improving processes and customer service have a hard time breaking out of this tradition. In spite of wholeheartedly adopting his seven habits, they are still recommending individual competitive rewards to get more participation from workers and more recognition from top management.

SEPARATE RECOGNITION FROM COMPETITION.

In every hospital where I facilitate focus groups, one common theme is sure to come up. "We need more recognition from our leaders." Or "We never hear our manager tell us when we do something good, only when we don't do something right or when we don't do enough." Or "We never feel appreciated for how hard we work."

People who exemplify the values of the organization and do the special things that generate customer and employee loyalty *should* be recognized. But recognition is not dependent on competition. Linking recognition to competition is a notion from our high-school days when we were in an independent reality. Competing for recognition is not what employees are talking about. They are hungry for appreciation, not contests. They want a word of encouragement, not to become teacher's pet. Why is it hard to see that you can have one without the other? I believe it's because of the "top honors" and "dean's list" syndrome that has been such a potent, and justifiable, part of the conditioning we received during our educational experience. It's hard to break out of well-established paradigms.

Many hospitals have adopted a caught-you-caring recognition system, which has been shown to increase expressions of appreciation and praise dramatically. Essentially it provides a handy card to recognizing any employee's efforts to provide special service or go above and beyond job expectations. So far, so good. But I have seen three variations on this basically good idea that are useless or counterproductive.

1. The cards are recorded and tracked so that rewards can be given, preferably by top management, to the people getting the most cards. (Remember the airline attendant?) I have already addressed the negative consequences of attaching competitive rewards to something like this.

2. Anyone can give a card directly to an employee whenever the giver sees something worth recognizing or appreciating. But what good is a card in this case? Can't the giver of the compliment just say thank-you whether or not they have a card? Besides, employees are not saying that their peers are not showing appreciation. They are saying that their *managers*, whose opinions are so important, are the ones who are so stingy with recognition.

3. Kits with cards and tokens are given to managers, who are encouraged to give them to employees that he or she "catches" doing the right thing. Again, what does this do, besides remind managers that they need to praise people when they do a good job? Not much, because managers who are stingy with praise will be stingy with cards and tokens. Nothing significant will change and managers will soon go back to their normal behaviors. In a year the program will be finished.

The system of recognition that I like—and have seen still in full operation and working beautifully after 10 and even 15 years—goes like this: Boxes (like suggestion boxes) with compliment cards are placed conspicuously in key locations, such as by the elevators and in waiting rooms. Anyone can use them, patients or employees. Someone is assigned to collect them at least once a week (more often if possible), and deliver them to the president in a small hospital or to the appropriate vice presidents in a large hospital. Top management reads all compliment cards and adds a note of thanks or just a signature indicating it was noticed. The cards are then routed through the chain of command to the employee. Presidents or vice presidents might select a couple of cards once in a while to deliver personally by hand. No prizes are given. The integrity of the employee's intrinsic motivation is

Management has to stay involved because the cards keep
hey can't opt just to quit reading them. And when the card is
the employee feels the rush of appreciation, made more
powerful because the appreciation arrives through management, not as
direct mail from the giver of the compliment.

A program like this is self-renewing and will go on successfully
forever as long as someone keeps collecting the cards and sending them
through management. That's because there is no reason to game the
system for rewards or leave it to individual managers to keep it going,
and the only motive for both giver and receiver is sincere appreciation.
Since recognition is never at the expense of somebody else, there is no
rivalry. And since there is no extrinsic reward, there is no cause for
cynicism about people's motives. People want to be appreciated for
doing the right thing, not given a prize. If I stop to help someone
change a flat tire, I am not looking for a reward and almost certainly
don't want money for my kindness, which would demean my motives.

EXTRINSIC REWARDS CAN DESTROY INTRINSIC MOTIVATION.

Several years ago I helped a hospital get a recognition program going. I
had warned the steering committee about the dangers of trying to
attach rewards to the system. I guess not all managers were warned, or
some did not see what was wrong with a little incentive once in a while
to get more of what you want from employees. The director of the
emergency department was disappointed in the lack of compliment
cards put in the box in the emergency area. She tried to encourage her
employee team to compliment each other more, but only a few more
cards came in. Finally she decided to offer a tiny reward. Surely there
could be nothing wrong with a small reward. So she told her employees
if a person filled out a compliment card, she would give the receiver a
free Pepsi.

What do you think happened? Did this director get more
compliments in the box? Of course she did. The box was stuffed with
compliments every day. Isn't this what she wanted? Yes. Well, if she got
more of what she wanted, why did she pull the plug on the offer within
a week? And when she did, why was the group up in arms? "What! No

more Pepsi? Well, just see if we put any compliments in the box now!" The cynics won the day. But worse, the cynics destroyed everyone's impulse to show appreciation, even when it was genuine.

The steering committee chairperson called me to find out how to rescue the recognition system that had turned into a joke in the emergency department. I told her it could not be rescued. One of the unintended consequences of offering a reward is that you can never take it back, because rewards quickly become seen as entitlements. People's attitude is, "You told us if we did this we would get that. Now you're taking that away. Why should we continue to do this?" In an astonishing reversal of desired outcomes, rewards can actually extinguish intrinsic motivation and with it the values the reward was supposed to encourage in the first place!

The story is told of an old man who was an expert in human motivation and behavior. He liked to work in his garden in the afternoon when kids were heading home from school. One day a couple of boys came by and yelled some insults at the old man, laughed, and ran away. The next day they did it again. This kept up for several days, and the group was growing and getting bolder. The old man ignored them, knowing that one way to extinguish an undesirable behavior is to ignore it because attention is a potent intrinsic reward. But the boys were having too much fun and getting plenty of attention from the other kids. The insults didn't stop.

The old man also knew that extrinsic rewards can often extinguish intrinsic motivation, so he came up with another plan. The next day when the boys came by, the old man spoke to them and said, "I have gotten to where I look forward to your insults everyday. And just to show that I am serious, tomorrow, whoever comes up with some really good insults will get a quarter. The next day the boys hurled their most outrageous epitaphs. Sure enough, they each got a quarter. The second day even more boys showed up and got quarters. Just think, they could get paid for having fun! On the third day there was a large crowd joining in, so the old man had to tell them, "Look, this crowd is getting too big. I can't afford to give you all quarters, so from now on I will just give you a penny per insult." The boys were indignant. "If you think we are going to do this for a penny, you're crazy," they said and refused to insult the old man again.

THERE ARE SERIOUS FLAWS IN FORCED CURVE MERIT PAY.

When I was a manager, I knew it was important to give frequent and accurate performance feedback to those who reported to me, but I felt my judgment would be seriously undermined by any system that forced me to grade each of my people on a curve that was then linked to pay increases. After recruiting the very best and getting rid of some poor performers, I had built a great team of high achievers. Their spirit of teamwork was crucial to getting the work of our department done. Each one performed a different task requiring different skills, but peak performance could come only from pride in their workmanship as a member of a high-performing team. To be forced by an arbitrary system to give some a higher raise than others whether it could be justified or not would be ludicrous and demoralizing. A typical example might be that an organization decides to give a 3-percent increase across the board as a raise for employees, allowing managers to hit that average by giving differing amounts from 1 percent to 6 percent, depending on the evaluations of a subordinate's performance. The problem comes when the system replaces the manager's judgment by demanding that some get less so that others can get more.

Pay for performance has a certain ring of truth and seemingly unassailable logic to it. Why should people be paid the same if they do not perform the same? Doesn't it demoralize the hard workers and encourage laziness when you give everyone the same increase in pay? Executives like Jack Welch, formerly of General Electric, placed a great deal of stock in this view of human motivation, carrying it to the extreme of *requiring* managers to fire and replace at least 10 percent of their employees every year, whether they wanted to or not.

If all individual jobs were identical, and had a direct link between individual performance and profit, this practice would not be the problem it creates where teamwork is essential. A person milling six machine parts an hour ought to get more than one who mills only four parts an hour. Hence we have piecework compensation. There are certainly many jobs that lend themselves to direct comparisons of output or income creation. Pay for performance started with them and appears to be more effective with them. As Ed Lawler writes in *From the Ground Up*:

> An individual pay-for-performance system does not fit an organization that is designed around processes and teams and that emphasizes the importance of lateral relationships and cooperation. Individuals who need to cooperate and help each other should not be put in a position of competing for the same rewards.[4]

What about nurses in a hospital? Are they not part of processes and teams with lateral relationships dependent on cooperation? And think of the variation in performance that is beyond their control. Every patient is different. No two situations are alike and individual care cannot be standardized as on an assembly line. Even patient flow cannot be controlled. Physicians can have radically different ways of doing things and make differing demands on individual staff members. A dozen departments must work closely with the patient-care team to deliver maximum results for each individual patient. About the only thing that comes close to a standardized system is charting. Should a nurse manager base the pay for performance on how well the paperwork is done because that is a fairly objective and individual activity? If we believe patient perceptions are vitally important, we have a problem with wide variations in perceptions, measurements, and comparisons. Then there is the effect of the nurse on the morale of the nursing team. It is vital too. Would we want a system that ignores what is subjective and rewards only what is objective? If the system lends itself to favoritism and accusations of unfairness, how effective is it?

In my case, one of the areas under my responsibilities was a creative marketing department that was so good it regularly ran away with awards that made big advertising agencies jealous. Each member of our creative staff had a different job to do but was an essential part of a synergistic team. Who should get the bigger raise? Ann, the receptionist who makes people feel welcome and cared for and would cheerfully do any task asked of her? Kevin, the copywriter who regularly writes great headlines and attention-grabbing lead paragraphs? Ani, the art director who consistently comes up with eye-catching designs and layouts? Kent, the coordinator who communicates regularly with the client and keeps the job on track with all the other projects that must be worked on at the same time?

Let's say my company insists that I give some less in order to give others more, but I believe that they are all of superior value and work ethic. After all, I didn't hire them on the curve. I didn't think I needed some weak ones in order to reward the better ones. In fact I hired each one from the top end of the bell shaped curve in the first place. In a pay-for-individual-performance system I could give only a median raise if I rated them all equally excellent. On the surface this seems fair, except that if 3 percent is the mid-range number, it says "You are barely average" to an employee. These talented people are all high achievers. Any one of them would be at the top of his or her class in a group of people doing the same thing. Their walls, which are lined with trophies, plaques, and awards, are proof that they have the talent. So are the results of their marketing efforts. How demeaning it would be to rate them all as average when they have worked with dedication and achieved a stature and recognition far above average. Nothing I can think of could sap their energy and sabotage their team spirit quite like being told that if I give one an "A," it has to come from somebody else who gets dropped to a "D"—or give everyone a "C." Worse still is that with the grade comes a difference in pay! Where is the logic or fairness in that? And how long could I keep such talented individuals if they felt unappreciated by their organization with no sensible justification based on their actual work? What would this do to their energy and motivation? To their self-confidence? To their morale? To their self-esteem? To their relationship with each other? To their relationship with me? The negative consequences of this arbitrary system can be disastrous. It's a system that creates one winner and five losers. To the one winner it will feel like a reward. But to the five losers, it will end up feeling like a punishment. Does that make it a system of rewards or punishments?

DISNEY DOES NOT RELY ON COMPETITIVE MERIT PAY.

Since I had come to believe that individual pay for performance or merit pay based on a normally distributed curve was the norm in American companies, it surprised me to find out that employees at Disney were not rewarded in a competitive system. Instead, everyone got raises based on longevity. About 10 percent, mostly top executives and department heads, did get bonuses based on predetermined goals, but annual raises for frontline cast members and their supervisors encouraged synergy, longevity, and cross-functional learning instead of competition.

When I learned this, I asked our teaching team if we shouldn't mention this to our hospital groups when they come to the three-day seminar we were preparing. The consensus was that it would raise too much controversy to bring it up since the hospital picked to represent the "Disney Way" as a showcase hospital maintained a pay-for-individual-performance system. If a question was asked, we could mention it, but we would not make it a key point in "Disney's Approach to Customer Service for the Healthcare Industry."

Personally, I felt this was a mistake. To me, the difference between a culture characterized by subjective performance evaluations coupled with competitive individual rewards is significantly different from one in which people are not put through such a demoralizing process that is fraught with secrecy, suspicion, politics, accusations of favoritism, and the inability to explain why one person receives more than another. I doubted that hospitals would ever be able to achieve the level of service and teamwork so evident at Disney without changing the compensation system to one that is more like Disney's. To me, this is not something with a minor influence on corporate culture.

In the division of Disney where I worked, each fulltime cast member wrote up a personal development plan. This plan was reviewed periodically with the person's manager. The cast member would evaluate his or her own progress and indicate areas for improvement and personal growth. The conversation and modifications to the plan were a shared effort with the manager, seen as a supporter and coach to help the cast member reach his or her own goals within the context of the team's goals.

183

I see nothing inherently wrong with using a bonus system, as Disney does, to prioritize goals for managers and the organization as a whole. As long as these bonuses are achievable and within the circle of a manager's control, or if all the managers are working together, they are probably useful.

DEMING ASSAILED INDIVIDUAL PAY FOR PERFORMANCE.

In the early eighties, I became acquainted with the writings of W. Edwards Deming, the father of the global quality movement who is credited, along with J.M. Juran and Peter Drucker, with teaching a bottom-up management philosophy that helped turn Japan's factories into the most productive in the world–and with the highest quality to boot! Deming's teachings assailed the traditional American management system of arbitrary individual competitive pay for performance.

Anyone with even a modicum of knowledge about the quality movement and its basic principles has heard of or seen a reenactment of Deming's famous red-bead demonstration. Most people think it's a demonstration of variation, a fundamental concept in Deming's quality control. But, though it does illustrate the impact of systems variation on individual performance, most quality instructors do not know the context of his demonstration. It is found in chapter 3 of his seminal book *Out of the Crisis*, which launched the quality revolution in America. The title of this chapter is "Diseases and Obstacles." Here is where he spells out his "seven deadly diseases" in American management. The red-bead demonstration is under the third disease, clearly stated as: "evaluation of performance, merit rating, or annual review." Here he assails American management's penchant for merit pay, individual pay for performance, and management by objectives. The red-bead illustration shows that most employees are victims of variation in processes and do not have enough control over them to be singled out for competitive merit pay. Here is how strongly Deming spoke against the practice of the competitive-performance review and merit-pay process:

Management by fear would be a better name, someone in Germany suggested. The effect is devastating. It nourishes short-term performance, annihilates long-term planning, builds fear, demolishes teamwork, nourishes rivalry and politics. It leaves people bitter, crushed, bruised, battered, desolate, despondent, dejected, feeling inferior, some even depressed, unfit for work for weeks after receipt of rating, unable to comprehend why they are inferior. It is unfair, as it ascribes to the people in a group differences that may be caused totally by the system that they work in...

Merit rating rewards people that do well in the system. It does not reward attempts to improve the system.[5]

Much has been written about the success of Deming's ideas and philosophy in Japan. In the United States, however, it has not been nearly so successful, although it has been almost universally adopted. At first this discrepancy was blamed on the diversity of the American workforce. Japanese companies, it was surmised, had a homogeneous culture with an innate work ethic and discipline that American workers lacked.

But then the Japanese showed they could do the same thing in American factories with American workers. By bringing in just a few executives at the top of the organization and changing the management systems, especially eliminating pay for individual performance and empowering teams, Japanese managers got the same incredible performance in America that they got in Japan. The difference, it turns out, is not in the *ethnic* culture, but in the *management* culture. Command and control structures, pay for performance, and management by objectives, assailed by Deming, were too deeply embedded and fiercely defended to be changed in most American manufacturing plants.

Western managers were enamored with the statistical charts and tools to better measure quality, but they could not turn substantial power and decision making over to process teams, the very strength that fuels exceptional performance. Instead of educating workers to take ownership and think and act for themselves, they second-guessed the recommendations of teams, instilled more "carrots" and "sticks" to maintain a culture of compliance and competition, and sapped the energy of intrinsic motivation with compensation systems that made people feel resentful instead of supported. No wonder Deming had such strong words against these systems of management that stifled the potential of turned-on workers. He knew that his ideas could take root only in the rich soil of empowered teams, not the unyielding ground of compliance and autocratically administered rewards. Luckily for the world, the Japanese were willing to listen.

PAY FOR PERFORMANCE IS ROOTED IN BUREAUCRATIC STRUCTURES.

Pay for individual performance or merit-pay increase was an extension of the point-factor system that has been so popular with companies steeped in traditional management style. Every job in the organization was pegged to a job description that spelled out knowledge requirements, working conditions, problem-solving skills, responsibilities, etc. Points were assigned to each of these criteria, which in turn determined the base pay for every job. This point-factor base pay was linked to an annual merit increase that was determined by an individual's performance appraisal. Finally the supervisor was forced to sort and rank evaluations on a normally distributive curve so that some performers got a higher percentage of the pie at the expense of others on the team who had to get less. When performance could be objectively measured, this was not such a problem. But in areas in which performance could not be judged objectively and was based on teamwork, this system wreaked havoc on morale and overall unit performance.

It is not my purpose to examine the history or the intricacies of the system, which probably determines 80 percent of American workers' pay. But I can certainly see how the system sustained a command-and-control culture. Bureaucracies grow out of top management's distrust of the ability of managers and supervisors to make decisions, including those about employee performance and compensation. The point-factor system and accompanying merit pay based on individual performance created the illusion of a perfect system by putting workers in precisely defined jobs and comparing them to other people. The arbitrariness of the system left little room for manager discretion or judgment. Unintended, of course, is the consequence that it also discourages employees from taking initiative and performing tasks outside their rigid job descriptions. This, in turn, provides little motivation for teamwork and collaboration. Workers become focused only on their own jobs instead of the quality of the product or service produced by their team, which decreases commitment, enthusiasm, and pride–all compelling motivators.

CAPITALIZE ON THE SUPERIOR POWER OF INTRINSIC MOTIVATION.

When extrinsic rewards become the focus of an organization's attempt to motivate the work force, the result is a culture of hierarchy and compliance. It creates a work environment of competition, fear, and defensiveness. No wonder the results are less than stellar and employees report a general feeling of low energy and morale.

In chapter 7, which is on imagination, I asserted that compliance is the weakest of all motivations because it does not tap into the power of our intrinsic desire to constantly do better. If I am spending my energies on covering my backside, not making any mistakes, or being envious of rewards given to others, there's not much left in the well for me to go to for personal growth. And this applies to managers as well.

Tom Werner, former president of Florida Hospital, circulated a memo to all his direct reports and asked us to describe the characteristics we most desired in reporting to a CEO. After we had returned our answers, he compiled a list and circulated it as a performance-evaluation form for our final approval. He told us he would like our evaluations on his performance in meeting our expectations. After our final review, we began to get these annually. They were sent to the secretary of the board of directors so our boss would not know who said what. Then the board chairman would go over the composite evaluation with him. He encouraged us to be candid, because only then would they be useful for his own self-improvement.

To me this was a demonstration of servant leadership. But it was also a demonstration of intrinsic motivation to improve, because there was no compensation attached to the results. He was asking subordinates to help him improve by sharing their honest perceptions. I'm sure Tom Werner hoped all his direct reports would follow his example and seek honest feedback from their subordinates also. But it didn't happen. Few vice presidents have the self-confidence to do it, and few corporate cultures are that open to upward evaluation without intimidation.

It is popular in many companies to do 360-degree evaluations in which managers are evaluated by their subordinates and peers, as well as their superiors. The idea sounds great. Jack Welch says he wished he had made his managers use them much sooner in his tenure as CEO of General Electric. When compensation is tied to the scores, however, honest feedback is thwarted. Managers know how to game the results. They know how, in subtle and not-so-subtle ways, to make sure employees are intimidated into giving high marks. Since culture follows structure, we may adopt an excellent feedback tool on the one hand and have a compensation structure on the other hand that renders its real purpose (self-improvement) useless. When that happens, we have a culture of fear that measures to impress, not to improve.

COMPETITIVE PAY FOR PERFORMANCE RENDERS COACHING USELESS.

The best possible performance feedback system is one that is driven by the intrinsic desire to improve, which we all have if it is allowed to rise to the surface and not be distorted by extrinsic considerations. Leadership seminars have expunged the word "boss" and extolled the word "coach" to describe the ideal manager. Yet management structures in the pay-for-performance model are antithetical to ideal coaching.

When I take a tennis lesson from my coach, Charlie O'Brian, I want criticism so much I am willing to pay for it. Imagine that: a subordinate asking—even paying—for criticism! Calling the evaluation process in most organizations "coaching" is a misnomer. It may be a form of supervision, but it is not coaching. The true coaching experience happens when a subordinate *wants* constructive feedback and *wants* to learn so he or she can do a better job. However, when the evaluation session is forced on an employee so that pay can be adjusted according to how one compares to others in a competitive environment, the most helpful element of the coaching model is destroyed. Threats and bribes make us conform but they do not make us receptive to criticism, even if we call it "constructive criticism." We get defensive. A defensive person is not open to learning. If every time my tennis coach tried to change part of my form I became resentful, argumentative, and defensive, what learning would take place?

THERE ARE FIVE QUESTIONS TO ASK YOURSELF.

By now the pay-for-individual-performance approach has been largely discredited as a de-motivational disaster, and stories about companies that have abolished it and achieved legendary results abound in the literature. It is not within the scope of this book to prove the case to a skeptic for removing competitive rewards as motivators. I have simply given my conclusions on the matter with a few observations, especially the fact that Disney has not used the practice through all its years of growth and excellence.

To anyone who is still skeptical, just look inside yourself and answer these five questions:

1. If there was no bonus at stake, or if everyone got the same bonus for achieving collective goals, would your work deteriorate?

2. If your manager points out to you that you missed some of your goals, would you work any harder to improve if your manager docked your pay or your bonus?

3. If other people on your team were to get 100 percent of the bonus but you didn't, would you feel motivated or de-motivated? Inspired to excel or depressed? Rewarded or punished?

4. If you were to get less than 100 percent of the raise that others got, would you feel more like helping out the whole team or competing with its individual members to prove yourself, even if it is at their expense?

5. Would you be likely to be more honest or less honest with your boss about your performance and areas for improvement if there was a financial reward or punishment attached to the evaluation?

Probably the most thorough examination of this topic has been done by Alfie Kohn in two books: *Punished by Rewards* and *No Competition*. Kohn and his researchers have collected and examined all the research that can be found on the effectiveness of rewards and competition in various environments. The results are astonishingly congruent, given the passion of opposing sides on the subject.

For those readers who like sports analogies for work teams, and believe that this kind of thinking is contrary to the seemingly self-evident fact that competition is the essential force behind athletic success, keep in mind the difference between internal individual competition between team members, and a team's competition with other teams. John Wooden, arguably the greatest college basketball coach of all time, often said, "A player who makes a team great is more valuable than a great player." Although he coached some great individual stars like Kareem Abdul-Jabbar and Bill Walton, he placed higher value on their character and teamwork than on their individual skills, and showed he could win national championships with teams without superstars. He was the one who invented the now-common practice of insisting that any player who scores must acknowledge, with a nod or hand-signal, the player who set up the score with a good pass. His basketball players also knew that he was more pleased in games where four or more players had scored in double digits than when one player got conspicuously more points than his teammates.

ENSEMBLE IS A BETTER METAPHOR.

I think most of our idea of competition comes from trying to compare work teams to sports teams. This is unfortunate, because the essential element in sports is winner-take-all competition. That is not the essential element in work teams where my work affects other teams whose success depends on me. If the next team down the line loses because of my poor work or our careless hand-off, then we all lose. Winner-take-all is a defeating strategy at work, not a winning one. Even if we take the element of competition out of work and try to compare ourselves to sports teams, what kind of sports team are you going to choose for your model? Are you like a baseball team where every player has a specific job to do and is expected to protect his turf? Or are you like most basketball teams where the ten other players are expected to get the ball to the one or two superstars who get all the credit when the game is won, and none of the blame when the game is lost? Or maybe you like football for a team analogy where one person calls all the plays and players are expected to execute the play exactly as told or get fired if they don't. Personally, if I had to choose a sports team analogy, I think I would pick volleyball–where everybody gets to serve and play every position even if they are better at some than others. In volleyball success depends on setting each other up and on how well they cover for each other. But when have you ever heard of volleyball used as an analogy for work teams? Which brings up one more blindspot: we prefer team analogies with sports that are the most masculine and where success comes from being the most physically dominating.

Better than sports analogies for work, are analogies in keeping with *work as theater* that we described in Chapter 6. In an orchestra or jazz group, or with actors in a play, they work every bit as hard as any sports team to achieve excellence, but there is no competition, no winners and losers, and no prize other than the praise of the audience. These groups are so different from sports teams, we call them something else–ensembles. To succeed, an ensemble doesn't even need a leader as long as they all know the script or musical score. They may improvise and take turns starring in solo moments, but they never stray from the intentions of the script or the score. But it is in the rewards where they are the most different. The only reward for an ensemble is not in beating another ensemble, or in winning a trophy, but in how they are perceived by the audience. When the audience applauds, they have their reward. And likewise, when our patients applaud, we have ours.

1. Steven R. Covey, *The Seven Habits of Highly Effective People: Restoring the Character Ethic* (New York: Simon & Schuster, 1990), p. 206.
2. Ibid.
3. Ibid., p. 230.
4. Edward E. Lawler, *From the Ground Up* (San Francisco: Jossey-Bass Inc., 1996), p. 211.
5. W. Edwards Deming, *Out of the Crisis* (Cambridge, Mass.: Massachusetts Institute of Technology, 1982), p. 102.

CHAPTER 10

CLOSE THE GAP BETWEEN KNOWING AND DOING

What separates Disney from all the other wannabes in the experience economy, or in the service economy too, is not Disney's unique knowledge about what customers want. It is Disney's consistency in the day-to-day execution of universally shared values and commonly desired behaviors. Like Pete Sampras, one of the greatest male tennis players of all time, Disney does all the same things everyone else in their field does, but Disney does them more consistently, especially under pressure and over a longer period of time—the qualities that separate champions from the rest of the pack.

This gap between knowing and doing is not easy to close in an organization in which managers have never been held accountable for the results of satisfaction surveys of patients and employees. Somehow administrators keep hoping that a different consultant will have the secret. They keep trying over and over to close the knowing-doing gap without changing the deeper things that cause the gap and keep it stubbornly in place. They are like a talented tennis player constantly looking for the coach that will have the secret to winning without hard, grueling work. Maybe there is a special shot. Maybe there is a secret strategy. Maybe there is a miracle diet. But more than anything, it is hard work.

I'd like to examine five major traps to closing the gap.

P #1: Expecting trainers and committees to transform the ̲ure. My single greatest frustration, in the beginning with my own organization, Florida Hospital, and virtually every client since, is the persistent, almost implacable belief that the main secret to Disney's success is its two-day training program, "Disney Traditions." The right service standards and training, it is believed, will effect a transformation in the culture. To keep the momentum of the program going, committees are installed to disseminate customer-service information and how-to knowledge. Using the model in Figure 10.1, let me try to demonstrate the fallacy of this approach and the vital missing piece in transforming and maintaining a culture of experience excellence. In this model there are three requisite components (we'll add a fourth later):

Figure 10.1: Performance Model (Part 1)

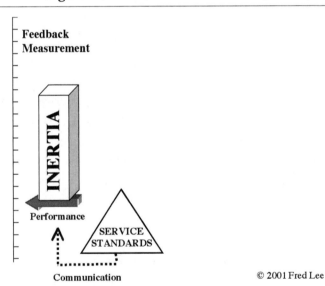

© 2001 Fred Lee

1. Employee performance, shown here as being under the weight of the inertia of habit.

2. Some form of feedback data measures the perceptions made by this performance.

3. Widespread improvement is accomplished, so the theory goes, by setting service standards and communicating them through a training program that will inspire more consistent performance.

If these training programs have outstanding trainers and the content receives high marks from the attendees, there is often a bump in the scores that appears to validate the training effort. Feedback data begin to show an upward trend, and optimistic administrators hope the trend will continue. The trouble is, it *never* does. As the curve flattens or begins to descend, committees are set up to figure out what is happening and how to keep employees motivated. In our model, committees are part of the triangle labeled "service standards." They are an extension of the work trainers are doing and, more than likely, include trainers in their composition. Committees churn out job descriptions with courtesy behaviors. They write scripts to improve first impressions and communication. They set up compliment and suggestion boxes. They order the *Fish* video and pass fishes out to each other. They publish letters from delighted customers. They disseminate patient-satisfaction scores. They hire mystery patients and circulate the report of opportunities for improvement. They work very hard. But nothing much happens to those intractable patient-feedback scores.

Look at the model again and notice that the program's influence is shown as a dotted line. At best a great program has some influence (dotted line), but *absolutely zero solid-line authority over those who attend.* That's right: zero line authority. With no authority over employee behavior, how can the inertia of poor habits ever be overcome? With no authority trainers and committees are left only with cajoling as their main technique to effect change. And we expect them to accomplish this in a one-time seminar for a day or even half a day! Look how unsuccessful we are with attempts to lose weight and keep it off when we are highly motivated. How do we expect people who are not particularly motivated to change their behavioral habits by going to a seminar? And even the motivated ones get quickly discouraged when they go back into the same work environment with the same indifferent spirit and same unconcerned manager and vice president.

Let's add the missing element to our model (Figure 10.2). Leadership. Only directors and managers have authority over performance and can effect change.

Figure 10.2: Performance Model (Part 2)

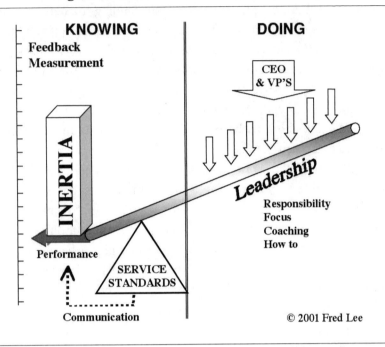

This model puts the four major elements in the right relationship. It does not show that programs are not important or should be abolished. It doesn't diminish the role of inspired committees or motivated employees. It simply shows that reading vision statements, knowing patient expectations, hearing stimulating stories, and learning communication and attitude skills are the *fulcrum*, not the *lever* for improvement.

Whenever trainers teach the SHARE program, which we developed at Florida Hospital and have improved through the years for other hospitals, there is one question that comes up over and over: "Are our managers going to pay any attention to this?" The second most asked question is "Are the doctors going to go to this program?" Any reader of this book knows exactly what they are trying to say. "This is all very well and good, but unless our managers buy in, role-model it and require it, this will not become standard practice." Hourly employees themselves know what it takes, even if their managers do not or wish otherwise.

During the two-day Disney Traditions, every cast member at Disney learns that exceptional service will be expected on the job. It is his or her chance for *knowing* what is going to be required. What happens when that cast member gets to his or her stage area? If it were a typical hospital, nothing much would happen that has anything to do with what was taught in the program on patient loyalty. The themes that sounded so important, the vision and core values, the stories that were so moving, the courtesy standards, the communication skills, are rarely referred to again. But at Disney the program is just the beginning of a daily obsession of directors, managers, and supervisors who turn *knowing* into *doing*. Responsibility and accountability occur in one's work area, not at the feet of trainers. Nor can they be maintained by a steering committee.

TRAP #2: Hiring a service-excellence coordinator. As committees pick the low-hanging fruit by tackling things like parking and signage problems, writing courtesy standards into job descriptions, designing reward and recognition systems, scripting first impressions, offering phone etiquette training, setting up boxes for compliments and suggestions, posting patient fan letters, and making sure patient-survey results are visible, it soon becomes obvious that they need someone to coordinate and maintain all these activities. Taskforces are wonderful for generating ideas and starting things, but they are not intended to maintain systems and programs. In the beginning all the initial work is absorbed by the taskforce members, but nobody believes they have taken on a permanent job or have installed a permanent committee. As the committee runs out of ideas and individual members want to hand off their tasks, it is natural to propose a coordinator who can coordinate all the activities started by the committee.

But a coordinator is in the same position as the program and the committees were in the first trap: no line authority over any department or employee. The coordinator may be able to do the clerical work on things like suggestions and compliments. He or she may be able to coordinate and even teach the orientation classes in service excellence for new employees. Recognition and reward programs can be folded into the coordinator's job description. But as we have shown, he or she is on the knowing side, not the doing side in our performance model.

It is only by the leverage of leadership that patient satisfaction and loyalty scores can be raised. Only managers and supervisors are responsible for performance and have the authority to hold people accountable. None of the coordinator's activities will do that.

There are two major ways to improve performance: through systems and through behaviors. With no systems and with no employees under the direction of the service-excellence coordinator, how can there be any significant improvement in satisfaction scores? I am not against a coordinator for the activities started by committees, but it is generally thought that the coordinator will somehow be able to raise and maintain satisfaction scores. That is unrealistic. As a vice president once said so bluntly and correctly, "My people do what I tell them to do. If I pay attention to something, they will. Otherwise they won't." That is the stark reality in a nutshell.

TRAP #3: Thinking more knowledge will close the gap. How much information or knowledge does a manager need in order to find ways to make internal processes serve the internal customer better? How much knowledge do nursing managers need before they can require courtesy, notice the lack of team spirit, deal with negative attitudes, reduce turnover, and role-model compassion in dealing with patients? The constant search for more knowledge is an insidious trap that sidetracks many administrators when they don't see much significant change in organizational performance.

In figure 10.2 there is a dividing line separating those activities that are about *knowing* and those that are about *doing*. Teaching does not qualify as doing, because it is simply part of learning. On the doing side of the model, there are four primary activities that help departments exercise leadership in doing: taking responsibility for walking the talk, focusing on what's most important in the customer's experience, coaching others, and doing the things that win the hearts of customers and staff.

We have developed a national appetite for knowledge, as all the books on leadership and model organizations can attest. We call this "the information age" and tremendous resources are being allocated to "knowledge management" and creating "the learning organization." But very little of all this knowledge actually gets transformed into action.

It is a trap to believe that knowledge is a force for change or action. Unfortunately it is not. Action comes about by *doing*, not by knowing or thinking or planning or listening or talking. In fact the most effective ways of doing are learned from trial and error, not necessarily from knowing *how* before one starts to *do*. As Jeffrey Pfeffer and Robert Sutton write in their book *The Knowing-Doing Gap, How Smart Companies Turn Knowledge Into Action*:

> One of the most important insights from our research is that knowledge that is actually implemented is much more likely to be acquired from learning by doing than from learning by reading, listening, or even thinking. Spend less time just contemplating and talking about organizational problems. Taking action will generate experience from which you can learn.[1]

Organizations are even poor at learning from themselves. Have you ever heard of anyone with a turnover problem making an effort to learn from someone else in their own organization who has an exceptional record of keeping good employees? Even when such a person reads several books on the subject and attends numerous seminars on retention, nothing is likely to change. According to Pfeffer and Sutton, Americans are famous for knowing and not doing. In Japanese companies the concept draws a blank, because the Japanese learn by doing, and if you are learning by doing there is no gap between knowing and doing.

TRAP #4: Letting assessment substitute for action. Measuring feedback is one of the elements in our performance model. I believe every department should be tracking feedback from its customers, internal or external. But feedback does not in itself cause actions to be taken on the feedback. Most hospitals have patient-satisfaction feedback, but few, if any, managers do anything with it or because of the information in it. When problems become conspicuous and distort the delivery systems, the normal reaction is to do a formal assessment of the problem and write a proposal for its solution. Yet how many of these activities turn into action that eliminates the problem or improves the system?

It seems quite normal for a hospital to beef up its information systems for patient satisfaction and loyalty when they launch a service-excellence initiative. Scores are refined. Efforts are made to achieve a higher return rate. Each care unit is given its own set of scores. Every physician starts to get the evaluations and comments on his or her behavior. The cycle time for information from the survey is shortened to have something closer to real-time information. Notebooks are beautifully organized and made more readable for top management. All this work usually entails adding another person to do the added clerical work to present the information in a timely, graphic, colorful way.

But assessment is not action. It is just another thing on the knowing side of our model, not the doing side. What emergency department needs more assessment to tell them that the waiting time between coming in the door and actually seeing a physician is the most important time measurement? Or that the speed with which they respond to the patient's pain is a critical satisfaction metric? Or that the number of patients who walk away without seeing a physician is a sign of dissatisfaction? Where serious response problems exist, knowing more about them will not improve the metrics. Even knowing how to improve the systems, which is well documented in the literature, doesn't mean they will actually do it.

Focus groups can provide valuable insights into customer needs and wants or identify barriers to excellence, but they are not a substitute for action either.

TRAP #5: Permitting managers to stall indefinitely with "How?" questions. I am convinced, after years of consulting, that this is the most harmful of all the traps. The first four have some good things in them. They are not harmful. They are simply on the side of the equation that is about knowing instead of doing. But the How? trap will sabotage the entire effort, quite possibly forever.

Since the How? trap is so detrimental, perhaps it should have been number one in this chapter. But it comes last because that is the order in which it finally shows itself, if it ever does, as a problem. After about three years of cycling through the first four traps, senior management begins to think that improving the scores is impossible and gives up. For three years their managers have successfully played the How? game, and top management is worn out from trying to answer that question by hiring consultants, assigning books to read, sending managers to seminars, convening focus groups, refining satisfaction-feedback information, running contests, writing mission statements and core values, posting service standards, setting up steering committees, changing job descriptions, implementing a recovery system for disgruntled patients, etc.

Since the average tenure of a hospital CEO is less than five years, middle managers can pretty well outlast all the service-excellence initiatives. By the time the administrator leaves, inertia will have won the day. Any new initiatives from a new administrator will be met with cynicism because the organization is now well inoculated against the virus of service excellence. And even if a determined leader at the top goes ahead, the old guard know they can stonewall their way with their tried and true smokescreen, "Show us *how* to do it in our department. Heaven knows, I'm a big supporter of our mission and core values and customer service. Just tell me *how* to do it, *how* to measure it, *how* to get people involved, *how* much it will cost, and my department will be there 100 percent. Are there any good seminars I can go to or good books I can read? Can I go visit some other hospitals and see how they do it? Maybe we should all go to Disney for a few days. What about getting a consultant who can really show us *how* to do it? The last one was a pretty good motivator but wasn't very specific about *how* to do it in *our* hospital with our run-down facility, labor shortages, awful payor mix, low wages, piles of paperwork, fierce competition and an overly demanding public with unrealistic expectations. We're not Disney, you know." Chalk up another win for inertia.

"HOW?" IS NOT ACCEPTABLE IN A CRISIS.

Holy Cross Hospital in Chicago was the first large, urban hospital I know that received national exposure for going from the lowest quartile in patient satisfaction to the very top among the 400, at that time, or so hospitals in the Press Ganey database.

They did not embark on finding the right consultants or books or seminars or site visits to other organizations. For them it was the simple fact of survival for the board and the CEO, and consequently the entire management team. Being at the bottom can do that. It can create a real crisis not felt in hospitals that are already pretty good compared to their competition.

Liz Jazwiec, who was the director of the emergency department at Holy Cross, has found a lucrative market for her story. Everyone wants to hear her tell about going from being the worst emergency department in patient satisfaction to one of the best. What is interesting to me is that Liz would not have done what she did by listening to or reading about anyone with a story like hers. She readily admits that she had successfully stonewalled any efforts to be held accountable for patient-satisfaction scores in her department. She was the expert in emergency services, not administrators, and certainly not consultants. She played the How? game as a smokescreen to cover up her lack of "want to." When Mark Clements, her boss, said, "There's no reason that you can't be as good as Disney World at customer service," she thought he was completely out of touch with reality.

"You want to see Disney World?" she would say, "I'll show you Disney World. Come down to my department some Friday night about one A.M. We've got Adventure Land. We've got Never Never Land. We've got Tomorrow Land. We've got Fantasy Land. We've got the whole thing for you."

When the rest of the hospital went from the 14th percentile in patient satisfaction to the 75th percentile in six months, the emergency department was still at only the 8th percentile. Liz says she took that as validation that their department was the only department doing the real work of saving lives and stamping out disease. Obviously everyone else had time for that service fluff, but her people didn't. But Mark Clements was not pleased. He gave her two choices, either believe in the goals and follow the program or leave. "Unless you drastically change these scores in 90 days, you're fired," he said. In the meantime he moved her replacement into her office. Without a choice, she did it, pulling off what she considered to be impossible.

Whenever anyone asks Liz Jazwiec how she caught the vision of service excellence and where she learned the leadership skills to make such spectacular improvement in only a couple of months, she admits that she did not read any books or go to any seminars. "I was nearly fired twice," she tells them candidly.

The gap between knowing and doing is a fallacy because managers already know all that is needed to achieve satisfaction in the services they have control over. More knowledge will not lead to action if the manager does not desire it at a deep level of commitment and intensity. Peter Block, a major author, consultant, and speaker in leadership circles, has captured the essence of this problem in his recent book, *The Answer to How Is Yes*. "Asking How? is a favorite defense against taking action."[2] He goes on to enumerate a family of How? questions that he equates with stalling tactics.

How long will it take?

How much does it cost?

How do you get them to change?

How do we measure it?

How have other people done it successfully?

Liz Jazwiec did not get anywhere by claiming not to know the answers to any of these questions, and her CEO did not permit her to stall indefinitely with How? questions. He simply said, "Do it, or I'll get somebody who will."

Baptist Hospital in Pensacola, Florida, was another hospital in the bottom quartile of patient satisfaction. The situation was deemed a serious crisis that demanded an immediate turnaround. Then they heard about the amazing story of Holy Cross Hospital in Chicago and Al Stubblefield, COO of the Baptist system, asked Quinton Studer from Holy Cross, to be the new CEO of Baptist Pensacola. Most hospitals have heard of Quint and the rest of the story. Baptist went on to have the highest patient and employee satisfaction scores in the Press Ganey database, and won the coveted National Malcolm Baldridge Award in 2004. They have hosted hundreds of hospital administrators and managers who make the trek to Pensacoloa to find out how they do it. Their story will soon appear in a book entitled *The Baptist Health Care Success Story: Creating a Culture that WOW's* from Wiley Publishing.

Baptist Hospital is a popular mecca for managers stuck in the How? trap. It's easy to believe that hospitals are not enough like Nordstrom or the Ritz Carleton or Disney to transfer best practices. Surely Baptist Hospital holds the answers. After all it's a real hospital. But with many years of watching this game, I doubt that one in a hundred visitors will do anything significant from a site visit. One of my friends went to Baptist and heard the "Baptist Story." A manager had made a particularly impressive presentation. My friend was awestruck by the amount of hard work and time it took to stay focused on patient-satisfaction scores and keep them at the top. After the presentation she ran into the manager in the hallway and complimented her on the presentation. "How in the world do you find time to do all those things?" she asked.

The manager replied candidly, "If I didn't, I'd be fired."

ACCOUNTABILITY IS NOT CONTINGENT ON BEING TOLD HOW.

As long as managers can stave off accountability under the guise of getting more information, many of them will. It's human nature. The reason customer and employee satisfaction so often escape accountability is that they are rarely framed as life or death requirements in the same way we frame cost containment and clinical quality. Baptist and Holy Cross did and the result has proved that service accountability is possible.

When department heads are told to cut 10 percent of their department's salaries, they don't have the luxury of stalling by claiming they don't know how to do it and need time to study it first or to visit other places that can show them how. I have never heard a CFO say, "We can't hold them accountable for reducing costs unless we can show them how to get the work done with 10 percent less personnel." Yet that same CFO will let managers use that excuse in patient satisfaction and employee retention.

The truth is that we hold people accountable all the time without telling them how to do what is required. Our problem is rarely with not knowing how. Our problem is with wanting to badly enough to break our habits of indifference, dependency (waiting to be told how to), and

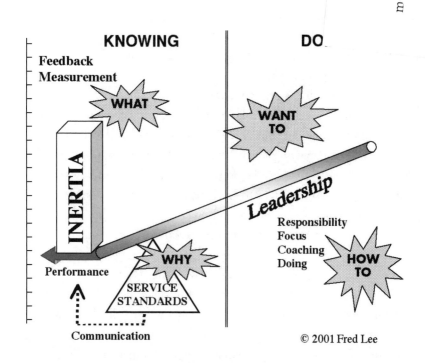

© 2001 Fred Lee

---

insecurity. If we cannot inspire it in ourselves, someone else will force it upon us if it matters enough. The best managers don't wait for that.

In Figure 10.3 each component answers a different question.

Every manager needs to know the answers to the What? questions and convey them to employees:

What matters most to the customers of our department?

What makes a difference in the way our department is perceived?

What do we, as a team, want to accomplish together?

What do we need from each other to do our best work?

What do we need from a manager (me) to excel?

What should we be measuring for feedback?

What will we do with feedback information?

very manager also needs to strengthen the service-excellence message contained in the mission statement and core values, the Whys?:

Why is patient loyalty so important?

Why doesn't customer satisfaction equal customer loyalty?

Why is my job important?

Why is my attitude and courtesy important?

Knowing is a vital part of learning and sharing a vision of what we want to create together. But "how" questions are on the doing side of the model. As in playing tennis, we learn how by doing. There is no other way. We can read books on tennis techniques and strategies. We can get a good tennis player to show us how he or she does it. We can watch players on TV for hours and analyze every stroke. But only by doing will we ever be able to learn how to do it. We may make mistakes but mistakes actually teach us more than our successes. Charlie, my tennis coach, often plays mini-games with me. He plays the points at my level of play, but every time I make a mistake, he makes me pay for that mistake by showing me what happens when I do that against an opponent at my level. If I go down the line when I should go crosscourt, he shows me what will most likely happen, and I learn more from making that mistake than I learn by all the telling me what to do in the world.

Finally (or maybe we mean firstly), it takes desire to accomplish a dream, the "want to" of motivation. Wanting to is on the doing side of our model because without wanting to, we certainly will never implement the difficult "how-to" work of actually leveraging performance. It takes a strong "want–to" to give a manager the energy to figure out how, and implement it with the full understanding and support of his or her staff. If you are a competent and self-confident manager, and want to badly enough, you will find the way. The great managers, like all great performers, will make it look easy.

The Healthcare Advisory Board had one word to describe the difference between hospitals that receive high patient-loyalty scores and those that don't: *hardwiring*. When responsibility for satisfaction and loyalty is hardwired into every manager's accountabilities, then courtesy gets hardwired into every employee's performance evaluation. As Liz Jazweic says, "We do what we are held accountable for doing."

This chapter has made a case for a culture of compliance. However I do not believe a culture of compliance is the ultimate goal for an organization. Obviously compliance can only take an organization so far. It can take a poor culture and make it better, even good. But to go from good to great, the culture will need to be a culture of commitment, not compliance. Commitment means that the vast majority of employees take ownership, and are just as commited as leaders to the success of the organization. They desire excellence for its own sake, not to get rewards or avoid sanctions. Like a good citizen, they make self-sacrificing decisions every day for the good of the whole. They take pride in their organization and they are its most active promoters. They are jealous for the reputation they have in the community.

So why the emphasis on leadership, accountability, and compliance? Because I believe compliance is a necessary transitional stage from an inconsistent, chaotic culture, to a culture that is self directed and can be trusted with the jewels of the company–patient loyalty. Much like children in a family, we often must go through the stage of adolescence, where one is partially free to make choices, but must still follow the rules of the household. To leave the dependency culture of childhood and get to the interdependency of adult citizenship, adolescents must endure a culture of compliance.

At Disney one cannot tell the difference between a culture of compliance, which it certainly is, and a culture of commitment, which it also is. Like a family, when everyone is operating in sync and functioning at peak effectiveness, how can you tell if they are obeying the rules because they want to or because they have to? In the final chapter of this book, the conclusion, I will offer some hints.

---

1. Jeffrey Pfeffer and Robert I. Sutton, *The Knowing-Doing Gap: How Smart Companies Turn Knowledge Into Action* (Boston: Harvard Business School, 2000), pp. 5, 6.

2. Peter Block, *The Answer to How Is Yes* (San Francisco: Berrett-Koehler Publishers, 2002), p. 11.

CONCLUSION

Have you ever worked very hard along side other people and absolutely loved every minute of it, even though you were physically exhausted at the end of the day? If so, what made it so enjoyable?

If someone were to ask me these questions, I would tell them about the summers when our family spent its traditional week at my wife's mother's house in Medford, Oregon.

My mother-in-law was in her eighties and lived alone on a small social security check. Her three daughters and their families would descend sometime in the spring and spend strenuous days planting a huge garden to give grandma another year of produce. We would paint what needed painting. We repaired things that were broken. One time we put new shingles on her roof. Another time, we put up grab rails where she had precarious footing, and a front porch banister as she became less steady on her feet. But what we all remember is the joy, the utter happiness we felt in hard work. Nobody needed a boss. We all pitched in where extra hands were needed. Someone went to the market. Someone cooked wonderful, wholesome meals, made more delicious by hearty appetites.

Children found plenty to do as they cheerfully joined in. They weeded the flowerbeds and washed windows and scrubbed floors without being bribed or coerced to do so. In fact, offering money would have diminished their intrinsic motivation–the fun of working with loved ones–that fueled all our efforts and brought pleasure in the hard work that made it possible for grandma to continue living in her little house on Peach Street. She was able to live alone there until she was 91 years old, when a fall required her to sell her home and live with one of her daughters, Sally.

With this personal metaphor in my mind, I would describe the perfect work environment as finding an unsurpassed level of joy in hard work with good friends, doing something important for someone else who cannot do it for themselves. What comes closer to this picture than being a caregiver in a hospital? The question is, how does one create such a team, and maintain such a spirit?

Dreams Motivate

I will never forget the tingling sensation of rapture I felt as I watched my television set on August 28, 1963. Martin Luther King Jr. was speaking to 200,000 people from the steps of the Lincoln Memorial in Washington D.C. giving one of the greatest speeches of all time. It has become known as the famous, "I Have a Dream" speech. Millions of Americans from all walks of life were stirred as they listened to a descendant of slaves say, "I have a dream that one day this nation will rise up and live out the true meaning of its creed: 'We hold these truths to be self-evident, that all men are created equal'...I have a dream that my four little children will one day live in a nation where they will not be judged by the color of their skin but by the content of their character." The words still echo in my mind and continue to inspire me when I recall them.

Martin Luther King Jr. did not say, "I have a strategic initiative." He did not say, "I have a plan." Somehow we know it would not have been very inspiring if he had. Plans and initiatives, and most mission statements, do not inspire people. It is articulating a dream that inspires commitment and motivation.

Carl Sandburg wrote, "Nothing happens unless first a dream." Certainly Walt Disney was primarily a dreamer of great dreams. His dreams eclipsed his artistic talent, but he was able to inspire talented people to share his dreams and make them a reality. When people are part of a team that is inspired by the same dream, they will do their own initiating and planning. A system of threats disguised as monetary rewards are not necessary, and will in fact undermine their spirit. These are the tools of uninspired leaders. And with these tools we can win people's compliance but not their hearts.

So start with your own dream by remembering a time when you loved working with other people. Analyze what made the experience so great. Then translate those principles into your current work environment by sharing that dream with your team every day.

If I were to take the personal metaphor for work I started v
spell it out, I would do it in a series of behavioral stateme
indicate the elements that must come together to create the dream. It
might look like this:

I dream of working in a department where…
    We all feel like friends
    Who find meaning in our work
    Together as a team with a shared passion
    To create the best experience for our patients (or customers)
    For the overall success of our organization.

I would then present these statements to the people who report to
me and have them share their thoughts. By taking each of the five
statements separately, we would have a springboard for important
conversations about what it would take to make that statement a reality.
For instance, the one that says, "Together as a team with a shared
passion," I might treat my staff like customers by asking them to
respond honestly to a series of probing statements they can complete in
as many ways as they wish:

About teamwork, I would ask the group in a staff meeting to complete:
    I want to work for a manager who…
    I want to work with coworkers who…
About passion, I would ask each individual to privately complete:
    I enjoy my work when…
    I wish there was less…
    I wish there was more…
    When I am not at work, I enjoy…

In order to track their impressions of teamwork, I would develop
two evaluation forms based on a synthesized list of the desires they
agree they care most about. One form would be used to evaluate me,
and the other form for them to evaluate each other. These could be
solicited on a quarterly basis at first. Then when it becomes obvious

that after making corrective adjustments we are achieving our dream of teamwork, they might be used less frequently.

For the keys to passion I would study carefully what each person disclosed about himself or herself. From their statements I would try to match people's personality to their work assignments better. And instead of managing everybody in the same way, I would look for the clues that tell me how each person prefers to be motivated and recognized. These individual responses also provide a nice framework for personal conversations that can probe for even better understanding of each person's special talents and preferences. Relating better usually means managing better.

This process of probing for information, having frank conversations, taking corrective actions, and getting feedback on performance, are the proven steps for continuous improvement in the things that cannot be measured statistically.

EXCELLENCE IS FUN.

Anything done at the level of excellence, or in the pursuit of excellence, is exciting and fun. Anything done at the level of mediocrity is discouraging and a real drag. Where there is low morale, we often make low pay or hard work the scapegoats. However, I suspect it is more often the dispiriting effect of poor team performance, finger-pointing negativity, and uninspired leadership.

The best way I know of to break this vicious cycle of poor performance that leads to low morale, that leads to poor performance, is to inspire a team to become better and better in an area they all believe is important. Let me repeat this notion to emphasize the universality of the psychological truth that anything done at the level of excellence is exciting and fun, and anything done at the level of poor to mediocre is boring and discouraging.

Although Walt Disney has been the example in this book, there would be no science, no technology, no discipline, no product of any kind, were it not completely fascinating and fun to somebody who became an expert, and worked hard at the level of excellence to present it to the world.

I remember how discouraging tennis was to me when I first took it up late in my life. As I watched others practice at a high level of competence, I knew at my age I would never be that good. The only thing that kept me at it was that jogging was even more boring than hitting a ball against a wall, or a ball machine, or a coach, no matter how poorly I hit. It wasn't until I had reached a certain level of competence that I started to really enjoy it. There was a time when I was sure I would never be able to have a decent serve. When I started playing doubles with guys older than I, they would move in to receive my serve, and then easily hit the ball pretty much anywhere. I will never forget the day when I noticed that they were actually stepping back for my first serve. It was exhilarating, and now I am so passionate about playing tennis, I could play it every day. As we get better at anything, we love it more. Hard work is never a drag when we love what we are doing. I love to work hard in a tennis lesson or a match—even to exhaustion. It is the improvement and the pursuit of improvement combined with proof of improvement that makes anything fun.

Nothing inspires like success. There is nothing like becoming excellent at something to meet our basic drive for competence, and feed our deep hunger for meaning and growth. This is the source of passion. Knowing and believing this truth about human motivation can make an ordinary manager a great coach. Learning to let go and allowing people to learn from their own mistakes and improve their own decision-making skills, will transmit the excitement to them.

HAVE THE RIGHT CONVERSATIONS WITH THE RIGHT PEOPLE.

I am convinced, as I pointed out in a previous chapter, that our problem is not with knowing how to do the things this book is meant to inspire. It is with having the right conversations with the right people in the right spirit. My hope is to use insights and observations from Disney to provoke thoughtful and candid conversations about the most important aspects of culture and work. A manager who does not have time for these vital conversations can only manage by coercion, because it is through openly expressed thoughts and feelings that we can uncover the hidden impediments to our dream.

Choose the Right Words with the Right Meanings.

Words are more than representations of thoughts. They actually shape our thoughts. Here are some words that have shaped my thoughts about leadership for many years, as they have probably shaped yours. And yet each of them gives us a connotation that I believe falls short in some important aspect. In order to change our thinking, we should probably change some words like:

Service
Leadership
Empowerment
Accountability
Starts at the top

If you have read this book, you already know what I want to say about some of these, and can probably guess the others. So consider this a review of some key concepts.

Service should be changed to experience. We are not at a patient's bedside to provide a service. We are there to provide a compassionate healing experience so the body can mend itself.

Leadership still implies a "leader" from whom most or all direction flows. In my metaphor for work at grandma's house, there was no designated leader. We all gave up a little of our own freedom to do as we wished, in order to help take responsibility for the success of the whole. That is the definition of citizenship, not leadership. Yes, "dispersed leadership," a popular theme today, is certainly in the right direction, and I am a great proponent of it. But with the word leadership, frontline employees usually think of its popular meaning. They are not schooled in the nuances of what the literature means by leadership. We may mean "leading by participation; everyone a leader." But what they still interpret from the word is "looking above for direction." So, why don't we rely less on a word with a double meaning, and rely more on a word like "citizenship" when we mean everyone can take charge and do what has to be done without being told?

Empowerment implies someone in authority conferring power on someone else. Unless the power is conferred, a person does not have it. Empowerment goes with the word leadership. A leader confers and removes power. But now that we have substituted the idea of citizenship for leadership, the traditional connotation of empowerment does not work. A better word to use with citizenship is ownership. In a democracy, the citizen takes ownership of the values that bind society and defines his own responsibilities in terms of them. We need employees who take ownership of the values that define a committed work culture in the same way that we need citizens who take ownership of the values of society.

Accountability also flows from leadership. The subordinate is accountable to the boss. But if we have citizens who have taken ownership of the cultural values, then accountability to someone in authority doesn't fit the paradigm. Accountability needs to be changed to responsibility. Citizens who take ownership will act responsibly. They give up some of their own freedom in order to take responsibility for the success of the whole.

Finally, if we have changed the leadership paradigm slightly, we need to get rid of the notion that it must "start at the top." The truth is, it can start anywhere. Remember the food service that introduced room service? That did not start at the top. Folks at the top need to encourage a culture of citizens who take ownership and responsibility, because ideally, it is citizens who come up with the ways in which the corporate culture can live out its dream of creating an unforgettable experience for patients and guests.

Do You Have A Story To Share?

I would enjoy hearing from readers. As a speaker and writer, I am interested in stories that illustrate the themes in this book. If you wish to share any of your ideas, insights or experiences, or contact me, I can be reached at <u>FredLee@PatientLoyalty.com</u>.